MCQs in Applied Basic Sciences for Medical Students
Volume 2

Dr Jonathan Fishman &
Dr Laura Fishman

MCQs in Applied Basic Sciences for Medical Students
Volume 2

Dr Jonathan Fishman &
Dr Laura Fishman

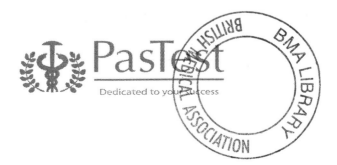

© 2006 PASTEST LTD
Egerton Court
Parkgate Estate
Knutsford
Cheshire
WA16 8DX

Telephone: 01565 752000

First Published

ISBN: 1 905635 15 X
978 1905635 15 3
A catalogue record for this book is available from the British Library.

The information contained within this book was obtained by the author from reliable sources. However, while every effort has been made to ensure its accuracy, no responsibility for loss, damage or injury occasioned to any person acting or refraining from action as a result of information contained herein can be accepted by the publishers or author.

PasTest Revision Books and Intensive Courses

PasTest has been established in the field of postgraduate medical education since 1972, providing revision books and intensive study courses for doctors preparing for their professional examinations.

Books and courses are available for the following specialties:

MRCGP, MRCP Parts 1 and 2, MRCPCH Parts 1 and 2, MRCPsych, MRCS, MRCOG Parts 1 and 2, DRCOG, DCH, FRCA, PLAB Parts 1 and 2.

For further details contact:

PasTest, Freepost, Knutsford, Cheshire WA16 7BR

Tel: 01565 752000 Fax: 01565 650264

www.pastest.co.uk enquiries@pastest.co.uk

Text prepared by Carnegie Book Production, Lancaster
Printed and bound in the UK by Athenaeum Press, Gateshead

Contents

About the authors   vi

Preface   vii

Mastering MCQs   ix

Abbreviations   xi

Section A

Mechanisms of disease   1

    The immune system in health and disease   3

    Medical microbiology   13

    Cancer biology   21

    Principles of pathology   31

    Section A – Answers   39

Section B

Therapeutics   113

Section B – Answers   123

Section C

Cellular biology and clinical genetics   143

Section C – Answers   155

Section D

Medical statistics and epidemiology   171

Section D – Answers   179

    Index   187

About the authors

Dr Jonathan M Fishman, BM BCh (Oxon), MA (Cantab), studied pre-clinical medicine at Sidney Sussex College, University of Cambridge, graduating in 2001 with a first class honours degree in Natural Sciences. He continued with and completed his clinical training at St John's College, Oxford and the John Radcliffe Hospital, qualifying in 2004. He is currently undertaking basic surgical training in London and his interests lie in teaching and medical education.

Dr Laura M Fishman, MB BS, BSc (Hons), is the twin sister of Jonathan Fishman. She qualifed in 2004 from Imperial College London with a first class honours BSc in Endocrinology. She is currently undertaking general medical training in London. She is keen to pursue a career in medicine and maintain an interest in undergraduate education.

Preface

More and more emphasis is being placed on multiple choice questions (MCQs) in the assessment of the medical school curriculum. The reasons for this are several fold. MCQs have the inherent advantage of being objective and unbiased, in addition to being comparatively easy to mark compared with conventional methods of assessment, such as short answer questions and essay writing. The rapid expansion in both the number of medical schools and the intake of students has led to MCQs becoming the assessment method of choice.

There are many MCQ books currently available. However, there is clearly a need for an MCQ series that deals with the 'early' or 'pre-clinical' years where the emphasis is on the applied basic sciences. A thorough grounding in the basic sciences is necessary, in order successfully to progress through the clinical school years. Indeed the importance of the basic sciences is highlighted by the emphasis placed on these in many of the postgraduate membership examinations that follow.

We have decided to dedicate an entire two volumes of MCQs to the applied basic sciences. This is not because we feel that the applied basic sciences are badly taught (although this may be the case in some medical schools!), but rather because we feel that many young medical students fail to appreciate the significance of learning about particular topics, or fail to make a link between the basic sciences and clinical practice.

The rationale behind this book is not only to provide practice in answering MCQs in the applied basic sciences, but also to bridge the gap between the applied basic sciences and clinical practice. Wherever possible we have endeavoured to correlate the basic sciences with clinical medicine. Not only should this make the basic sciences more enjoyable and retainable, but it will also help the young medical student to recognise and appreciate the importance of learning such material. If after working through these volumes medical students are better able to apply their basic scientific knowledge to clinical practice then we have successfully achieved our goal.

Jonathan Fishman and Laura Fishman

Mastering MCQs

The secret to passing any kind of MCQ exam is to practise as many questions as possible. Sitting in front of large textbooks will help to a degree, but it is important to get a feel for the type of questions that may appear in the exam and then to focus revision on reading around the questions. Whatever curriculum you currently follow, there will always be core questions that will be tested at the undergraduate level. We hope to cover those core questions.

Each question has five possible answers. One answer will be correct and the other four will be false (single best answer format). One of the first techniques in approaching these types of questions is to cover up the answers initially, read the question and suggest an answer. Then look for the answer in the options available. If the answer appears, you have a very high chance of being correct. You should check that the other answers are in fact incorrect, before selecting your final answer. If you are unable to answer the question initially, work your way down the list and start by eliminating those answers that you definitely feel are incorrect. Even if you are left with two possible answers you have a 50% chance of getting the correct answer by guessing, rather than the 20% chance that you started with. The exam is not usually negatively marked at the undergraduate level, so do not leave or miss out any questions.

If there are any questions that you are unsure of, asterisk that question so that, if you have time, you can come back to it at the end. One should also consider that certain words in the question can give you a clue to getting to the right answer in the exam. For example:

- 'Always' is, more often than not, always false in medicine.
- If the word 'never' appears, it is always never true.

Research has shown that changing your answer in the exam is neither good nor bad: if you have a good reason for changing your answer, then change it. It is a myth that people always change from 'right' to 'wrong', in that it is those incorrectly changed questions that you will remember and review after the exam. You will not remember the questions you changed from wrong to right!

Although everyone may tell you before the exam 'READ THE QUESTION', it is imperative to do so in the MCQ exam. Underline the key words, and do not be caught out, as so often people are, when the question says which of the following is false as opposed to being true! When you have finished the exam, make a final check that you have answered ALL the questions. Never forget to ensure that you have answered the last question and not forgotten to turn over to the last page.

We hope you enjoy the book and find it a pleasurable form of learning. All that is left to say is – Good Luck!

Abbreviations

5-HT	5-hydroxytryptamine (serotonin)
AAFB	acid–alkali-fast bacilli
ACE	angiotensin-converting enzyme
ACTH	adrenocorticotrophic hormone
ADH	antidiuretic hormone
AIDS	acquired immune deficiency syndrome
ATP	adenosine triphosphate
bFGF	basic fibroblast growth factor
BCG	Bacille Calmette–Guérin vaccine
BSE	bovine spongiform encephalopathy
Ca^{2+}	calcium ions
cAMP	cyclic AMP
CD	clusters of differentiation
Cl^-	chloride ion
CJD	Creutzfeldt–Jakob disease
CMV	cytomegalovirus
CNS	central nervous system
COMT	catechol-*O*-methyltransferase
CRP	C-reactive protein
DNA	deoxyribonucleic acid
EBV	Epstein–Barr virus
ER	endoplasmic reticulum
H^+	hydrogen ions
H_2O_2	hydrogen peroxide
HA	haemagglutinin
Hb	haemoglobin

HDL	high-density lipoprotein
HHV	human herpes virus
HIV	human immunodeficiency virus
HLA	human leukocyte antigen
HMG-CoA	hydroxymethylglutaryl-coenzyme A
HTLV	human T-cell leukaemia virus
Ig	immunoglobulin
IL	interleukin
K^+	potassium ions
LDL	low-density lipoprotein
LPS	lipopolysaccharide
MAO	monoamine oxidase
MHC	major histocompatibility complex
mRNA	messenger RNA
Na^+	sodium ions
NA	neuraminidase
NADPH	reduced nicotinamide adenine dinucleotide phosphate
NK	natural killer
NMJ	neuromuscular junction
NSAIDs	non-steroidal anti-inflammatory drugs
PCR	polymerase chain reaction
PG	prostaglandin
pH	$-\log_{10} [H^+]$
PKU	phenylketonuria
$P(o_2)$	partial pressure of oxygen
PPAR	Peroxisome proliferator-activated receptor
PPI	proton pump inhibitor
PTHrP	parathyroid hormone-related protein

Rb	retinoblastoma
RNA	ribonucleic acid
SD	standard deviation
SE	standard error
SLE	systemic lupus erythematosus
TB	tuberculosis
TNF	tumour necrosis factor
VEGF	vascular endothelial growth factor
VLDL	very-low-density lipoprotein
WHO	World Health Organization

Section A
Mechanisms of disease

The immune system in health and disease
Questions

1 The following are features of the adaptive (acquired) immune response:

○ A Acute inflammation
○ B Secretion of tears
○ C Natural killer (NK) cells
○ D Surface epithelia
○ E Self-/non-self discrimination

Answers on page 39

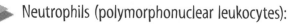

2 Neutrophils (polymorphonuclear leukocytes):

○ A Are the predominant cell type in chronic inflammation
○ B Have bilobed nuclei
○ C Have a lifespan of only a few hours in inflamed tissue
○ D May fuse to form multinucleate giant cells
○ E Carry out oxygen-dependent microbial killing by lysosomal enzymes

3 The germinal centre of a lymph node:

○ A Contains mainly T lymphocytes
○ B Contains Langerhans' dendritic cells
○ C Generates immunoglobulin (Ig)-producing plasma cells
○ D Is characteristically enlarged in established infectious mononucleosis
○ E Contains the cords and sinuses

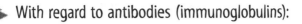

4 With regard to antibodies (immunoglobulins):

○ A Antibodies are produced by mast cells
○ B The antigen-binding region is located in the constant region
○ C Antibody class is defined by the structure of the light chain
○ D Diversity is partly achieved through somatic hypermutation
○ E Antibodies are composed of one heavy and two light chains

5 IgM antibodies:

○ A Cross the placenta
○ B Are characteristically produced in a secondary immune response
○ C Can activate complement
○ D Are usually found lining mucosal surfaces
○ E Are usually monomeric

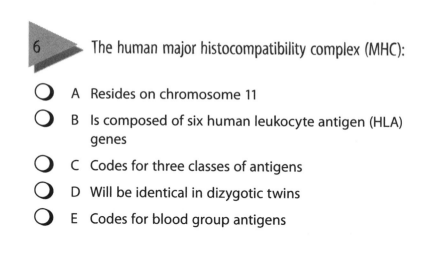

6 The human major histocompatibility complex (MHC):

○ A Resides on chromosome 11

○ B Is composed of six human leukocyte antigen (HLA) genes

○ C Codes for three classes of antigens

○ D Will be identical in dizygotic twins

○ E Codes for blood group antigens

7 With regard to the MHC:

○ A CD4 (helper) T cells recognise antigen only in the context of MHC class I

○ B Class II MHC is expressed on all nucleated cells of the body

○ C Class II MHC contains β_2-microglobulin

○ D Class II MHC presents exogenous antigens

○ E Class II MHC is expressed in low levels on the surface of dendritic cells

8 ▶ The classical pathway of complement activation:

○ A Starts with the activation of the C3 component
○ B Is activated by lipopolysaccharide cell wall constituents
○ C Is activated by IgA immune complexes
○ D Is activated by IgM immune complexes
○ E Is evolutionarily older than the alternative pathway

9 ▶ Which of the following cells are cytotoxic?

○ A CD4 T cells
○ B CD8 T cells
○ C B cells
○ D T helper 1 or T_{H1} cells
○ E T helper 2 or T_{H2} cells

10 ▶ With regard to the acute phase response:

○ A Bacterial endotoxin induces the acute phase response

○ B Exogenous pyrogens act on the liver to release tumour necrosis factor-α (TNF-α)

○ C The acute phase response is mediated through interleukin-10 (IL-10)

○ D Serum albumin levels increase during the acute phase response

○ E TNF-α decreases catabolic activity

11 ▶ Fever:

○ A Results from the direct action of micro-organisms on the brain

○ B Depends on the action of prostaglandins within the hypothalamus

○ C Is always maladaptive and serves no purpose

○ D Results only from infectious causes

○ E Is helped by the antipyretic action of aspirin as a result of boosting the immune response

12 ▶ The following are immunologically privileged sites except:

○ A Central nervous system (CNS)
○ B Skin
○ C Eye
○ D Uterus
○ E Testis

13 ▶ Type I hypersensitivity:

○ A Is caused by antigen reacting with IgM antibodies
○ B Results in mast cell degranulation
○ C Is characterised by the Arthus reaction
○ D Takes 48–72 hours to develop
○ E Is caused by the formation of antibody–antigen complexes

14 ▶ Type III hypersensitivity:

○ A Is mediated by specifically sensitised T lymphocytes
○ B May cause allergic rhinitis
○ C Is a feature of nickel sensitivity
○ D May occur in systemic lupus erythematosus (SLE)
○ E Is cell mediated

15 ▶ Hyperacute rejection:

○ A Is a cell-mediated response
○ B Occurs 48 hours after transplantation
○ C Can occur in autografts
○ D May be reversed by high-dose steroids
○ E May be minimised by blood group matching

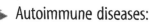

16 ▶ Autoimmune diseases:

○ A Are usually congenital

○ B Are overall more common in men than in women

○ C Arise when an immune response is mounted against a foreign antigen

○ D Result from a breakdown in immunological tolerance

○ E Are always humorally mediated

Medical microbiology
Questions

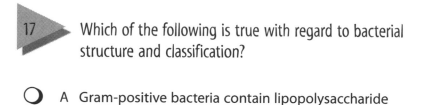 Which of the following is true with regard to bacterial structure and classification?

○ A Gram-positive bacteria contain lipopolysaccharide

○ B Gram-positive bacteria retain an iodine purple dye complex

○ C Gram-negative bacteria possess thicker layers of peptidoglycan than Gram-positive bacteria

○ D The endotoxin part of lipopolysaccharide is the O-antigen portion

○ E All cocci are Gram positive

Answers on page 55

18 Splenectomy increases susceptibility to which of the following organisms?

○ A *Streptococcus pyogenes*

○ B *Schistosoma haematobium*

○ C *Bacteroides fragilis*

○ D *Neisseria meningitidis*

○ E *Staphylococcus aureus*

19 Helicobacter pylori:

○ A Is a Gram-positive organism

○ B Is a known carcinogen

○ C Is present in about 5% of the population

○ D Is destroyed by the acidic environment present within the stomach

○ E Infection can be prevented through immunisation

20 ► Cholera:

○ A Is transmitted by the blood-borne route

○ B Is caused by infection with *Shigella sonnei*

○ C Is usually accompanied by marked mucosal inflammation and ulceration

○ D Is caused by a toxin that increases adenylyl cyclase activity

○ E Is caused by endotoxin

21 ► Hepatitis B

○ A Is an RNA virus

○ B Infection is more commonly cleared if acquired in childhood than later in life

○ C Is the second most common human carcinogen worldwide

○ D Is commonly acquired by the faeco-oral route

○ E Is effectively treated by hepatitis B immunisation

22 ► Human immunodeficiency virus (HIV):

○ A   Is a DNA virus
○ B   Contains RNA polymerase
○ C   Is transmitted by the faeco-oral route
○ D   Establishes persistence through antigenic variation
○ E   Principally targets CD8 T cells

23 ► With regard to influenza:

○ A   Influenza is caused by a DNA virus
○ B   The influenza virus belongs to the *Picornaviridae* family of viruses
○ C   Antigenic drift is responsible for pandemics
○ D   Mutations in the haemagglutinin molecule are responsible for antigenic drift
○ E   Influenza can be prevented by administration of a live vaccine

24 The pathogenicity of the tubercle bacillus is caused primarily by which one of the following?

○ A Ability to multiply within macrophages
○ B Delayed hypersensitivity reaction against the bacterium
○ C Direct toxic effect on host cells
○ D Effective antibody response
○ E Necrosis caused by expanding granulomas

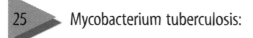

25 Mycobacterium tuberculosis:

○ A Is a Gram-negative organism
○ B Is an anaerobic micro-organism
○ C Typically affects the apical lung in post-primary tuberculosis (TB)
○ D Is treated with penicillin
○ E Is impossible to acquire after BCG immunisation

26 ▶ Tetanus:

- A Is caused by a Gram-negative bacillus
- B Is caused by an aerobic organism
- C Results from the secretion of exotoxin
- D Is caused by *Clostridium perfringens*
- E Is caused by bacterial invasion of the nervous system

27 ▶ Malaria:

- A Is caused by a virus
- B Is transmitted by the mosquito vector *Aedes*
- C Caused by *Plasmodium malariae* is the most virulent
- D May cause blackwater fever
- E Is effectively prevented by immunisation

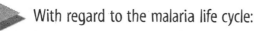

With regard to the malaria life cycle:

O A Sporozoites invade erythrocytes

O B Parasites may remain dormant in the liver as hypnozoites

O C Trophozoites invade hepatocytes

O D Schizonts are contained within the mosquito's salivary glands

O E Fertilisation and formation of a zygote occur in humans

29 ▶ With regard to schistosomiasis:

O A It is caused by a protozoan

O B The intermediate host is the sandfly

O C *Schistosoma mansoni* causes urinary schistosomiasis

O D Disease results from the immune response to schistosome eggs

O E It is treated with quinine

30 ► Prions:

○ A Are infectious micro-organisms

○ B Are destroyed by sterilisation

○ C Contain nucleic acid

○ D Cause disease by inducing mutations in the DNA of the host

○ E Are responsible for causing kuru in humans

Cancer biology
Questions

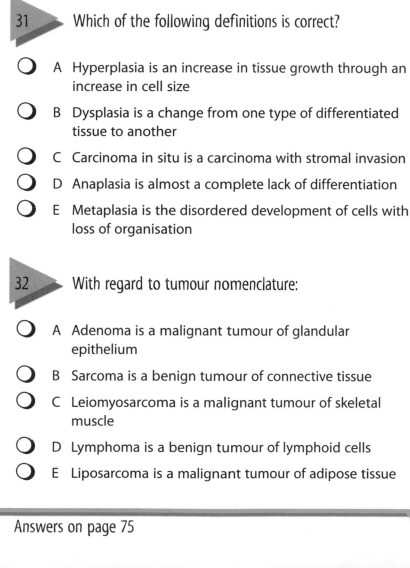

31 ► Which of the following definitions is correct?

○ A Hyperplasia is an increase in tissue growth through an increase in cell size

○ B Dysplasia is a change from one type of differentiated tissue to another

○ C Carcinoma in situ is a carcinoma with stromal invasion

○ D Anaplasia is almost a complete lack of differentiation

○ E Metaplasia is the disordered development of cells with loss of organisation

32 ► With regard to tumour nomenclature:

○ A Adenoma is a malignant tumour of glandular epithelium

○ B Sarcoma is a benign tumour of connective tissue

○ C Leiomyosarcoma is a malignant tumour of skeletal muscle

○ D Lymphoma is a benign tumour of lymphoid cells

○ E Liposarcoma is a malignant tumour of adipose tissue

Cancer biology – Questions

33 ▶ With regard to metaplasia:

○ A It is irreversible

○ B It is most important in the upper oesophagus

○ C Metaplasia in the bronchus involves a change from columnar to stratified squamous epithelium

○ D Metaplasia is harmless

○ E Barrett's oesophagus involves a change from glandular to stratified squamous epithelium

34 ▶ Which of the following is a defining characteristic of a malignant tumour?

○ A Increase in size with time

○ B Chromosomal abnormalities

○ C Presence of a pseudo-capsule

○ D Invasion beyond the basement membrane

○ E Well-ordered maturation

35 Which of the following are cytological features of malignancy?

○ A Hyperchromatism
○ B Pyknosis
○ C Karyorrhexis
○ D Decreased nuclear:cytoplasmic ratio
○ E Low mitotic index

 36 Carcinomas most often metastasise by which of the following routes?

○ A Bloodstream
○ B Lymphatics
○ C Transcoelomic
○ D Perineural
○ E Implantation

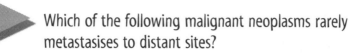

37 Which of the following malignant neoplasms rarely metastasises to distant sites?

O A Bronchial carcinoma

O B Breast carcinoma

O C Astrocytomas

O D Renal cell carcinoma

O E Melanoma

38 Sarcomas:

O A Are derived from epithelium

O B Are more common than carcinomas

O C Have a peak incidence in those aged less than 50

O D Metastasise more commonly by lymphatic than haematogenous routes

O E Have a long in situ phase

39 ▶ With regard to tumour kinetics:

○ A The smallest clinically detectable tumour is 1000 cells

○ B Tumour growth obeys gompertzian kinetics

○ C In most tumours the growth fraction is greater than 90%

○ D Tumour growth is characterised by contact inhibition

○ E The clinical phase of tumour growth is long compared with the pre-clinical phase

40 ▶ Angiogenesis:

○ A Is the process of programmed cell death

○ B Is highly dependent upon VEGF

○ C Is impaired when tumours grow larger than 1 mm^3

○ D Is always pathological

○ E Is inhibited by cytokines, in which granulation tissue is rich

41 An increased frequency of tumours caused by occupational carcinogen exposure has been proved in the following groups, except:

○ A Transitional cell carcinoma bladder and dye workers

○ B Scrotal carcinoma and chimney sweeps

○ C Mesothelioma and asbestos exposure

○ D Hepatocellular carcinoma and polyvinyl chloride exposure

○ E Malignant melanoma and sunlight exposure

42 For which one of the following tumours is there an association with Epstein–Barr virus (EBV) infection?

○ A Bronchial carcinoma

○ B Cervical carcinoma

○ C Burkitt's lymphoma

○ D Hepatocellular carcinoma

○ E Kaposi's sarcoma

43   With regard to oncogenes:

    A   They behave in a dominant fashion

    B   They encode proteins that regulate growth negatively

    C   *BRCA-1* is an oncogene implicated in breast carcinoma

    D   Transcription of oncogenes is dysregulated in normal cells

    E   Oncogenes are present only in tumour cells

44   With regard to tumour-suppressor genes:

    A   They encode proteins that positively regulate growth

    B   They behave in a dominant fashion

    C   Gain of function of tumour-suppressor genes results in neoplastic growth

    D   *p53* and *Rb-1* are tumour-suppressor genes

    E   *p53* normally functions as an anti-apoptotic factor

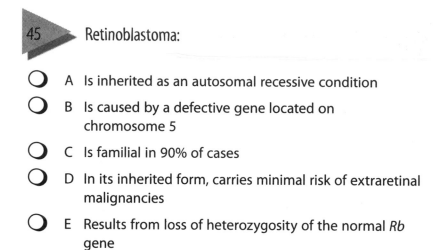

45 ▶ Retinoblastoma:

○ A Is inherited as an autosomal recessive condition

○ B Is caused by a defective gene located on chromosome 5

○ C Is familial in 90% of cases

○ D In its inherited form, carries minimal risk of extraretinal malignancies

○ E Results from loss of heterozygosity of the normal *Rb* gene

46 ▶ Lung carcinoma:

○ A Is the third most common cause of death from neoplasia in the UK

○ B Has rarely metastasised at the time of presentation

○ C May produce paraneoplastic syndromes

○ D Is most commonly the result of small cell (oat cell) carcinoma

○ E Is most commonly caused by asbestos exposure

47 Which one of the following is the most common intracerebral neoplasm?

○ A Astrocytoma
○ B Oligodendroglioma
○ C Meningioma
○ D Neuronal tumour
○ E Secondary carcinoma

 48 Which one of the following is the most common malignant tumour of bone?

○ A Chondroblastoma
○ B Giant cell tumour
○ C Osteosarcoma
○ D Chondrosarcoma
○ E Secondary carcinoma

Principles of pathology
Questions

 49 Apoptosis

○ A Is always a pathological event
○ B Involves the death of large contiguous areas of cells
○ C Is usually accompanied by inflammation
○ D May be seen in histological section
○ E Leaves a permanent clump of cellular debris

 50 Which of the following is true with regard to acute inflammation?

○ A The predominant cell type is the macrophage
○ B Inflammation is usually initiated by cell-mediated immunity
○ C Inflammation may last for many months
○ D Inflammation is intimately connected with the clotting system
○ E Inflammation is always the result of infection

Answers on page 93

51 The following are possible outcomes of acute inflammation, with the exception of:

○ A Resolution

○ B Chronic inflammation

○ C Abscess formation

○ D Amyloidosis

○ E Death

52 Chronic inflammation:

○ A Is always preceded by an acute inflammatory phase

○ B Usually heals by organisation and repair

○ C Is characterised by less tissue destruction than acute inflammation

○ D Usually results in resolution

○ E Involves neutrophils as the predominant cell type

53 The following inflammatory processes often involve granulomas:

○ A Lobar pneumonia
○ B Bronchopneumonia
○ C Tuberculosis (TB)
○ D Granulation tissue
○ E Ulcerative colitis

54 With regard to wound healing:

○ A Granulation tissue actively contracts
○ B Granulation tissue is defined by the presence or absence of granulomas
○ C Repair implies the complete restitution of normal tissue architecture and function
○ D In first intention healing the wound is unapposed
○ E Scar formation is absent in second intention healing

55 The following tissues are likely to regenerate after damage?

○ A Cerebral cortex

○ B Peripheral neurons

○ C Skeletal muscle

○ D Cardiac muscle

○ E Spinal cord

 56 Necrosis:

○ A Is a physiological or pathological process

○ B Involves single cells

○ C Is classically liquefactive necrosis in the brain

○ D Involves phagocytosis of the necrotic cells by adjacent cells

○ E Has caseous necrosis as the most common type

57 Which one of the following is the best definition of gangrene?

○ A Digestion of living tissue by saprophytic bacteria
○ B Digestion of dead tissue by saprophytic bacteria
○ C Gas production in dead tissue
○ D Necrosis of tissue caused by bacterial toxins
○ E Necrosis of tissue caused by ischaemia

58 Which of the following increases the risk of thrombosis?

○ A Immobility
○ B Thrombocytopenia
○ C Reduced blood viscosity
○ D An intact endothelium
○ E Heparin

59 An embolus:

O A Most often arises from a thrombus formed within arteries

O B Is the same as a thrombus

O C Caused by a thrombus is impossible to distinguish from a post mortem clot

O D Is always the result of a thrombus

O E Generally has a worse outcome than a thrombus

60 Ischaemia:

O A Refers to generalised tissue death as a result of toxins, trauma or vascular occlusion

O B Is synonymous with the term 'infarction'

O C Is an abnormal reduction of the blood supply to or drainage from an organ or tissue

O D Is always the result of vascular occlusion

O E Leads to a worse outcome in tissues with a collateral circulation

61 Acute myocardial infarction:

○ A Usually results from an embolus
○ B Always causes chest pain
○ C Induces acute inflammatory changes, maximal at 1–3 days after the infarct
○ D Is visibly apparent (on macroscopic examination) less than 12 hours after the infarct
○ E Involves replacement of the infarcted tissue by new cardiac muscle

62 Atherosclerosis:

○ A Is irreversible
○ B Most commonly occurs at branching points within the circulation
○ C Is a disease that primarily affects the tunica media of arteries
○ D Is accompanied by acute inflammation
○ E Is accelerated by hypocholesterolaemia

The immune system in health and disease

Answers

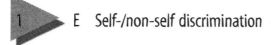

1 ▶ **E** Self-/non-self discrimination

Innate (natural) immunity comprises:

- physical barriers (skin, mucosal membranes)
- physiological factors (pH, temperature, oxygen tension, eg low pH of stomach inhibits microbial growth, commensal flora)
- protein secretions (eg lysozyme in saliva and tears, complement, cytokines, acute phase proteins)
- phagocytic cells (neutrophils, macrophages, NK cells)
- acute inflammation (including mast cells, histamine).

The two key features of adaptive (acquired) immunity are its specificity and memory.

The adaptive (acquired) arm of the immune response operates through both humorally and cell-mediated mechanisms and has a number of key features. Immunological tolerance is the exposure to self-components in fetal life that leads to a state of specific immunological unresponsiveness (anergy). In adulthood the adaptive immune system is therefore able to discriminate self from non-self, which is essential in preventing one's own immune system mounting a response against one's own tissues. It may become defective, resulting in autoimmune disease. Immunological memory is a feature of the adaptive immune response and is essential for the rapid response to subsequent exposure of antigens. This concept is central to understanding how vaccines work.

2 C Have a lifespan of only a few hours in inflamed tissue

Neutrophils are the most common type of leukocyte in the blood.

They are present in large numbers in acute inflammation, but in chronic inflammation macrophages predominate. They have multilobed, rather than bilobed, nuclei, with four to five lobes, rising to six to seven in patients with vitamin B_{12} or folate deficiency. The ability to fuse to form multinucleate giant cells is a characteristic of macrophages rather than neutrophils, and is classically seen in granulomatous conditions such as tuberculosis (TB).

The phagocytic ability of neutrophils plays a vital role in the host defence against infection. Microbial killing results from both oxygen-dependent and oxygen-independent mechanisms. The former is more important and depends on the 'respiratory burst', which follows activation of cell membrane NADPH oxidase by phagocytosis and results in the formation of powerful bactericidal agents (H_2O_2, superoxide anion and singlet oxygen). Oxygen-independent microbial killing is carried out by lysosomal enzymes, such as lysozyme.

The importance of oxygen-dependent bacterial mechanisms is illustrated by the congenital disorder chronic granulomatous disease. It results from inherited defects in the genes encoding several components of NADPH oxidase, rendering the patient susceptible to recurrent bacterial infections.

Neutrophils have a lifespan of only a few hours in an inflammatory lesion, sometimes less. A severe local infection quickly becomes a graveyard for thousands of neutrophils. Their content, especially enzymes, spill out and may cause additional damage to host tissues. This is known as immune pathology and is the price to pay for having a sophisticated immune system.

3   C   Generates immunoglobin (Ig)-producing plasma cells

The germinal centres of lymph nodes contain mainly B lymphocytes and follicular dendritic cells.

Follicular dendritic cells are able to trap antigen on their cell surface for long periods of time. They help to initiate a B-cell response to antigens entering the lymph node and play an important role in affinity maturation (a process that results in an increase in the affinity of the antibodies produced during the course of a humoral immune response). Follicular dendritic cells should not be confused with Langerhans' dendritic cells, which are professional antigen-presenting cells found in the skin. The cords and sinuses of a lymph node are situated in the medulla. The medullary cords are rich in plasma cells, whereas the sinuses are rich in macrophages. The paracortical zone (or inter-follicular area) is rich in T lymphocytes.

There is characteristically an expansion of the paracortex, rather than the germinal centres, in infectious mononucleosis (and many other viral infections) – so-called reactive hyperplasia. This manifests clinically as lymphadenopathy.

4 ▶ D Diversity is partly achieved through somatic hypermutation

Antibodies (immunoglobulins) are a heterogeneous group of proteins produced by plasma cells and B lymphocytes, which react with antigens.

All have a similar structure with two heavy chains and two light chains. In addition, antibodies are made up of variable and constant regions. The antigen-binding region is located in the variable region, whereas the complement-fixing and antibody receptor-binding activities are found in the constant region. The structure of the region of the heavy chain that is constant determines the class of the antibody (ie IgG, IgM, IgA, IgE). Although mast cells do not produce antibodies, they contain immunoglobulin receptors on their cell surfaces. As a result mast cells are able to bind pre-formed IgE on their cell surface, which plays an important role in allergy and anaphylaxis (type I hypersensitivity reaction).

Any individual has about 10^{10} different antibodies. This astonishing degree of diversity arises through four main processes:

1. The pairing of different combinations of heavy and light chains.

2. Recombination of V, D and J segments (VJ for light chains).

3. Variability in the joins of the recombined segments through imprecise joining by recombinatorial machinery and the addition of extra random nucleotides via terminal deoxynucleotide transferase.

4. Somatic hypermutation – a poorly understood mechanism for introducing mutations into V regions of activated B cells (antigen driven).

A malignant tumour of plasma cells may result in the overproduction of a monoclonal population of immunoglobulins. This is known as multiple myeloma.

5   C   Can activate complement

IgM antibodies are usually pentameric, whereas IgG is monomeric and IgA is usually found as a dimer linked by a J chain. IgM antibodies are characteristic of a primary immune response; IgG antibodies predominate in a secondary immune response.

IgM is an effective activator of complement when it has bound a specific antigen. IgA, rather than IgM, is found lining mucosal surfaces and is secreted into breast milk; IgA is therefore known as secretory immunoglobulin.

IgM cannot cross the placenta, whereas IgG can. The consequences of this are threefold: first, if IgM antibodies directed against infectious organisms are found in the fetal blood, they are an indicator of intrauterine infection; second, antibodies to ordinary ABO blood groups (anti-A and anti-B) are usually of the IgM type and hence do not cross the placenta; and third, because IgG can cross the placenta, whereas IgM cannot, it explains why rhesus haemolytic disease of the newborn is uncommon with the first pregnancy (the initial exposure to rhesus antigen evokes the formation of IgM antibodies). Subsequent exposure during a second or third pregnancy generally leads to a brisk IgG antibody response.

6 ▶ B Is composed of six human leukocyte antigen (HLA) genes

The human MHC is situated on chromosome 6.

There are six pairs of allelic genes (A, B, C, DP, DQ, DR). The human MHC will be identical only in monozygotic (identical) twins. There are two classes of MHC antigens: class I antigens are expressed on the surface of all nucleated cells, and class II are expressed only on the surfaces of cells such as antigen-presenting cells.

7 ▶ D Class II MHC presents exogenous antigens

There are two principal classes of MHC; both play an important role in antigen presentation and recognition by T-cells.

Class I MHC molecules are made up of one heavy chain and a light chain called β_2-microglobulin. Class II molecules do not contain β_2-microglobulin and consist of two chains of similar size.

Almost all nucleated cells of the body express MHC class I molecules on their cell surfaces. Hepatocytes express relatively low levels of class I MHC. This may explain why infection by certain hepatitis viruses (namely hepatitis B and C) or *Plasmodium* protozoa (the cause of malaria) commonly leads to a chronic carrier state in the host. Non-nucleated cells such as erythrocytes express little or no class I MHC; infection in the interior of red cells (such as malaria) can therefore go undetected. Class II MHC molecules are constitutively expressed only by certain cells involved in immune responses, although they can be induced in a variety of cells. Class II MHC molecules are richly expressed on the surface of dendritic cells.

The two classes of MHC are specialised to present different sources of antigen. MHC class I molecules present endogenously synthesised antigens (eg viral proteins). MHC class II molecules present exogenously derived proteins (eg extracellular microbes), which are first internalised and processed in the endosomes or lysosomes. Class I MHC molecules present peptides generated in the cytosol to CD8 T cells, whereas MHC class II molecules present peptides degraded in intracellular vesicles to CD4 T cells.

8 ▶ D Is activated by Igm immune complexes

The complement system consists of a large number of distinct plasma proteins, triggering a cascade of reactions where the activation of one complement component results in the activation of another. This amplifies the effector molecules of the complement system.

The main consequences of complement activation are the opsonisation of pathogens, recruitment of inflammatory cells and direct killing of pathogens. There are two principal pathways of complement activation: the alternative and classical pathways. The alternative pathway is the evolutionarily older of the two pathways but the classical pathway was discovered first, hence the term 'classical pathway'.

The alternative pathway is activated by the lipopolysaccharide of cell wall constituents, whereas the classical pathway is activated by IgM or IgG (but not IgA) that has bound to its specific antigen. Thus, in a transfusion reaction IgM from the recipient's blood binds to the incompatible donor red cells, leading to complement activation, haemolysis and acute renal failure. The alternative pathway starts with the activation of complement C3, but the classical pathway starts with the activation of complement C1 .

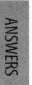

9 ▶ B CD8 T Cells

Lymphocytes can be divided into two main subtypes – T cells and B cells.

B cells (or plasma cells) secrete antibodies. T cells can be divided into two further subtypes: CD4 T cells and CD8 T cells. CD4 (helper) T cells can recognise antigen only in the context of MHC class II, whereas CD8 (cytotoxic) T cells recognise cell-bound antigens only in association with class I MHC. This is known as MHC restriction.

CD4 and CD8 T cells perform distinct but somewhat overlapping functions. The CD4 helper T cell can be viewed as a master regulator. By secreting cytokines (soluble factors that mediate communication between cells), CD4 helper T cells influence the function of virtually all other cells of the immune system, including other T cells, B cells, macrophages and NK cells. The central role of CD4 cells is tragically illustrated by HIV (human immunodeficiency virus), which cripples the immune system by selective destruction of this T-cell subset. In recent years, two functionally different populations of CD4 helper T cells have been recognised: T_{H1} cells and T_{H2} cells, each characterised by the cytokines that they produce. In general, T_{H1} cells facilitate cell-mediated immunity, whereas T_{H2} cells promote humorally mediated immunity.

CD8 cytotoxic T cells mediate their functions primarily by acting as cytotoxic cells (ie they are T cells that kill other cells). They are important in host defence against cytosolic pathogens. Two principal mechanisms of cytotoxicity have been discovered: perforin granzyme-dependent killing and Fas–Fas ligand-dependent killing.

10 ▶ A Bacterial endotoxin induces the acute phase response

The acute phase response is part of the innate (natural) immune system. Macrophages are exquisitely sensitive to the lipopolysaccharide (LPS) present in certain bacteria.

They respond by producing cytokines, notably TNF-α, and interleukins IL-1 and IL-6 (not IL-10, which can generally be thought of as an inhibitory cytokine). The aforementioned cytokines act on the liver to increase the concentration of many key serum proteins to aid the host defence response (such as C-reactive protein or CRP, serum amyloid protein, mannose-binding protein, fibrinogen, complement). CRP concentrations form a useful marker for detecting the presence (or confirming the absence) of inflammation or infection; this is a readily available laboratory test in the hospital setting. In addition, monitoring the trend in CRP values (as opposed to one-off values) provides the clinician with extremely valuable information as to whether the patient is getting better or worse.

Activation of the acute phase response is responsible for a number of different effects. First, it is responsible for the fever that may accompany a variety of different inflammatory and infectious states, through the action of IL-1 on the thermosensory centres in the anterior hypothalamus. Second, hepatic protein synthesis is diminished and the level of serum albumin decreases. This is an attempt by the body to conserve protein and is responsible for the hypoalbuminaemia that often accompanies many disease states. Third, TNF-α (cachectin) and IL-1 have catabolic effects and are responsible for the cachexia and anorexia seen in a variety of chronic inflammatory and infectious conditions. TNF-α is also believed to be responsible for the cachexia seen in malignancy (cancer cachexia). In this, TNF-α is produced by macrophages in response to the tumour, or by the tumour cells themselves. Finally, activation of the acute phase response is central to the pathogenesis of septic shock where excessive activation of the acute phase response leads to an overproduction of cytotoxic cytokines, resulting in a massive inflammatory reaction that may culminate in multiple organ failure and death.

11   B   Depends on the action of prostaglandins within the hypothalamus

Fever is brought about by toxins from micro-organisms that act on cells of the immune system to produce cytokines (including IL-1, IL-6 and TNF-α). It is the body's immune response to the invading micro-organism, rather than a direct result of the micro-organism itself causing fever.

The cytokines produced by the immune system act as endogenous pyrogens and act on the hypothalamus to generate fever, via the production of prostaglandins. Aspirin works as an antipyretic by blocking the enzyme (cyclo-oxygenase) that generates prostaglandins.

Fever also results from a variety of non-infectious causes, in addition to the infectious ones. Examples are various inflammatory conditions, connective tissue diseases, drug reactions and malignancies.

Fever is evolutionary advantageous; it inhibits the growth of some micro-organisms (most organisms grow well only in a narrow temperature range), increases the rate of production of antibodies, improves the efficiency of leukocyte killing and decreases the mobility of the host (thereby aiding recovery of the host and preventing spread of infection to other individuals). However, in some situations fever becomes maladaptive, resulting in hyperpyrexia, dehydration and death.

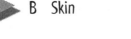

12 ▶ B Skin

Immunologically privileged sites are anatomical sites that are normally segregated from the immune system. Immunological privilege results from the effects of both physical barriers to cell and antigen migration and soluble immunosuppressive mediators such as certain cytokines.

Such sites include:

- CNS
- eye
- testis
- uterus (fetus)
- interior of red blood cells (one mechanism by which malaria evades the immune system).

Note that the skin is not an immunologically privileged site and is rich in Langerhans' dendritic cells.

By definition, immunologically privileged sites are sites in which immunocompetent hosts can maintain allogenic tissues without eliciting rejection. Thus HLA matching is not required for corneal transplants and the rarity with which such transplants are rejected has contributed to the considerable success rate of corneal transplantation. In addition, the immunologically privileged environment of the uterus may help to explain the mysterious lack of rejection of the fetus, which has puzzled generations of reproductive immunologists, but is obviously of compelling importance for the propagation of the species.

Damage to an immunologically privileged site can induce an autoimmune response, presumably because the adult immune system has never been exposed to the antigens sequestered in such sites. In other words, the immune system has not had the opportunity to become tolerant to such antigens. Thus, a breakdown in the blood–brain barrier may lead to multiple sclerosis (a chronic inflammatory, demyelinating condition of the CNS, resulting in multifocal white matter lesions separated in time and space), damage to the blood–testis barrier may result in infertility (an autoimmune reaction in a man to his own spermatozoa) and a trauma to the eye may result in sympathetic ophthalmia (where rupture of one eye results in the release of antigens, which triggers an autoimmune attack on both eyes).

13 B Results in mast cell degranulation

Hypersensitivity is a condition in which undesirable tissue damage follows the development of humorally or cell-mediated immunity. Gell and Coombs classified hypersensitivity reactions into four types. However, some also include a fifth type, as shown below.

Gell and Coombs' classification of hypersensitivity reactions:

1. Type I: mast cell degranulation mediated by pre-formed IgE bound to mast cells. Immediate (within minutes). Anaphylaxis, atopic allergies.

2. Type II: antibodies directed towards antigens present on the surface of cells or tissue components. Humoral antibodies participate directly in injuring cells by predisposing them to phagocytosis or lysis. Good examples are transfusion reactions, autoimmune haemolytic anaemia and Goodpasture's syndrome. Initiates within several hours.

3. Type III: formation of antibody–antigen complexes (immune complex mediated). Good examples are the Arthus reaction, serum sickness and SLE. Initiates in several hours.

4. Type IV: delayed type of hypersensitivity. Cell mediated. T

lymphocytes involved. Granulomatous conditions. Contact dermatitis. Initiation time is 24–72 h.

5. Type V: caused by the formation of stimulatory autoantibodies in autoimmune conditions such as Graves' disease.

ANSWERS

14 ▶ D May occur in systemic lupus erythematosus (SLE)

Type III hypersensitivity reactions are mediated by antibodies. Type IV reactions are cell mediated through specifically sensitised T lymphocytes. Nickel sensitivity is a type IV hypersensitivity reaction.

Allergic rhinitis is a type I hypersensitivity reaction. SLE is a type III hypersensitivity reaction where large amounts of immune complexes are created from nuclear antigens and antibodies. Latex allergies can be one of three types:

1. Irritant contact dermatitis (non-immune)

2. Allergic contact dermatitis (type IV hypersensitivity reaction)

3. Immediate hypersensitivity (type I hypersensitivity reaction or anaphylaxis) – what everyone worries about!

The immune system in health and disease – Answers

E   May be minimised by blood group matching

Hyperacute rejection is a result of the formation of preformed antibodies against the donor organ. It occurs within minutes of transplantation so that the surgeon can usually see the changes taking place as the anastomoses are completed.

The antibodies are usually directed against blood group antigens and so rejection can therefore be minimised by blood group matching. The blood groups and HLA antigens of autografts (tissue from the same individual) will be identical, so that hyperacute rejection will never occur in such circumstances.

No drug treatment can reverse hyperacute rejection; the only treatment is removal of the transplanted organ.

Transplant rejections can be classified into the following types:

- hyperacute: preformed antibodies (minutes to hours)
- accelerated acute: reactivation of sensitised T cells and secondary antibody response (days)
- acute: cytotoxic T-cell mediated with primary activation of T cells (days to weeks)
- chronic: antibody-mediated vascular damage (months to years, controversial).

Autoimmune diseases result from the direct attack by the host immune system against their own, or self, antigens (autoantigens), usually as a result of a breakdown in immunological tolerance.

These diseases are normally acquired, rather than congenital, and for some unknown reason they are more common in women than in men. The female preponderance is often taken to imply that sex hormones are involved in the pathogenesis.

The exact nature of the stimulus that triggers an autoimmune reaction is still unclear. The most plausible explanation is that certain exogenous agents (such as dietary factors, drugs or microbial agents), which share epitopes with self-antigens, stimulate an immune response against both themselves and the host tissues, producing tissue-damaging reactions. This is known as 'molecular mimicry'. However, genetic factors undoubtedly also play a role, eg autoimmune diseases are often associated with specific HLA types.

Although, in many cases, the precise combination of pathogenic mechanisms is not understood, either antibody or T cells can cause tissue damage in autoimmune disease.

Medical microbiology Answers

 17   **B**   Gram-positive bacteria retain an iodine purple dye complex

Micro-organisms can be classified into bacteria, viruses, fungi, protozoa and parasites. Bacteria can be classified according to the following:

- staining properties: Gram positive, Gram negative, acid fast, etc
- morphology: round (cocci), rods (bacilli), spiral (spirochaetes), comma shaped (vibrios), flagellated, possess capsules, etc
- oxygen requirements: aerobic or anaerobic, obligate or facultative
- ability to form spores: spore forming or non-spore forming.

In Gram-positive bacteria, the peptidoglycan forms a thick (20–80 nm) layer external to the cell membrane. In Gram-negative species the peptidoglycan layer is thinner (only 5–10 nm) but overlaid by an outer membrane. The principal molecules in the outer membrane of Gram-negative bacteria are lipopolysaccharides.

These structural differences form the basis of the Gram stain. Gram-positive bacteria are able to retain an iodine purple dye complex when exposed to a brief alcohol wash. Gram-negative bacteria have a smaller cell wall but a higher lipid content and, as a result, the alcohol washes away the purple dye. Gram-positive bacteria appear blue and Gram-negative bacteria are counterstained with a pink dye.

As a general rule:

- All cocci are Gram positive (except *Neisseria,* which causes meningitis and gonorrhoea).

- All bacilli are Gram negative (except *Clostridium* spp., *Mycobacterium* spp., *Listeria* spp., and the organisms that cause anthrax, diphtheria and actinomycosis).

The LPS in the outer membrane of Gram-negative bacteria is a complex molecule found nowhere else in nature; it is an important factor in bacterial survival in the mammalian host. It consists of three portions:

1. A lipid portion (lipid A) embedded in the outer membrane (the damaging endotoxin). As it is embedded in the outer membrane it exerts its effects only when bacteria lyse.

2. A conserved core polysaccharide.

3. The highly variable O-polysaccharide (O-antigen), responsible for antigenic diversity. It has been hypothesised that such structural variability is an attempt by the bacterium to evade host defences.

Endotoxins are not in themselves toxic (unlike exotoxins) but they can induce toxic effects as a result of their potent activation of the complement cascade, coagulation cascade and stimulation of the release of powerful cytokines (such as TNF-α and IL-1) from leukocytes. In overwhelming infections, the patient is said to suffer from endotoxic shock.

D   Neisseria Meningitidis

The spleen plays an important role in the removal of dead and dying erythrocytes and in the defence against microbes. Removal of the spleen (splenectomy) leaves the host susceptible to a wide array of pathogens, but especially to encapsulated organisms.

Certain bacteria have evolved ways of evading the human immune system. One way is through the production of a 'slimy' capsule on the outside of the bacterial cell wall. Such a capsule resists phagocytosis and ingestion by macrophages and neutrophils. This allows them not only to escape direct destruction by phagocytes but also to avoid stimulating T-cell responses through the presentation of bacterial peptides by macrophages. The only way that such organisms can be defeated is to make them more palatable by coating their capsular polysaccharide surfaces in opsonising antibody.

The production of antibody against capsular polysaccharide primarily occurs through T-cell-independent mechanisms. The spleen plays a central role in both the initiation of the antibody response and the phagocytosis of opsonised encapsulated bacteria from the bloodstream. This helps to explain why, after a splenectomy, the host is most susceptible to infection by encapsulated organisms, notably *Streptococcus pneumoniae* (pneumococcus), *Neisseria meningitidis* (meningococcus) and *Haemophilus influenzae*.

Understanding the above, one can quickly envisage what preventive strategies must be employed post-splenectomy. Patients are given relevant immunisations and advised to take prophylactic penicillin, in most cases for the rest of their lives. In addition they are advised to wear a MedicAlert bracelet to warn other healthcare professionals of their condition.

19 ▶ B Is a known carcinogen

Helicobacter pylori is a Gram-negative, micro-aerophilic, motile, spirally shaped bacterium that selectively colonises the mucus layer of the stomach and duodenum. About 50% of all humans worldwide are infected with the organism. However, it seems to cause disease only in a small proportion of those infected.

It is still unclear at present why this is the case, but it probably reflects differences in virulence among different strains, along with differences in the background genetics of the host, which affect their susceptibility to the organism.

It is now firmly established that *H. pylori* causes more than 90% of duodenal ulcers and up to 80% of gastric ulcers. The link between *H. pylori* infection and subsequent gastritis and peptic ulcer disease has been established through studies of human volunteers, antibiotic treatment studies and epidemiological studies. *H. pylori* is also a known risk factor for gastric adenocarcinoma and lymphoma. Indeed, *H. pylori* has been classified as a class 1 (definite) carcinogen for malignancy.

H. pylori is unique among bacteria in being able to survive within the acidic environment of the stomach. It achieves this by producing a urease enzyme that synthesises ammonia from endogenous urea, thereby buffering gastric acid in the immediate vicinity of the organism. The elaboration of urease by *H. pylori* forms the basis of the urea breath test, which may be used in the diagnosis of *H. pylori* infection. *H. pylori* is treated with antibiotic therapy. *H. pylori* eradication therapy (also known as triple therapy) usually consists of a proton pump inhibitor together with two antibiotics. At present, there is no known immunisation against *H. pylori*, although development of a vaccine against *H. pylori* would have the potential to prevent peptic ulcer disease and perhaps even gastric carcinoma.

D Is caused by a toxin that increases adenylyl cylase actvity

Cholera is caused by *Vibrio cholerae*, a Gram-negative, comma-shaped, flagellated bacterium. It is usually transmitted by contaminated water supplies, as deduced from the famous epidemiological work of John Snow in the 1850s; Snow was able to trace a cholera outbreak in London to a single water pump that had become contaminated with sewage. Removal of the handle of the water pump led to a dramatic reduction in the number of new cases of cholera.

The diarrhoea of cholera is caused by the action of an exotoxin or enterotoxin (not endotoxin) called cholera toxin. This toxin increases the activity of adenylyl cyclase, resulting in the massive secretion of chloride, sodium and water (so-called 'rice-water diarrhoea'). The watery diarrhoea may be so extreme that death may occur from dehydration and electrolyte imbalance. The mucosa is not invaded by the bacterium (in contrast to *Salmonella*, *Shigella* and *Campylobacter* spp.) so that mucosal inflammation is only slight and there is no ulceration.

Overall absorption from the gut remains intact so that oral rehydration therapy can replace massive fluid and electrolyte losses, reducing the mortality rate from 50% to less than 1%. Antibiotics (such as tetracyclines) are used as an adjunct to fluid therapy. Antibiotics diminish the duration and volume of the fluid loss and hasten clearance of the organism from the stool.

21 ▶ C Is the second most common human carcinogen worldwide

A third of the world's population are currently infected with the hepatitis B virus. Hepatitis B is a double-stranded DNA virus, usually transmitted haematogenously, by sexual intercourse, or vertically from mother to baby. Hepatitis A (not hepatitis B) is acquired by the faecal–oral route.

Infection during childhood leads to a high rate of chronic carriage of the virus, with only 10% of children clearing the virus. This chronic carrier state is associated with long-term complications in later life. Ninety per cent of adults, on the other hand, clear the virus, with only 10% becoming chronic carriers of the virus.

Hepatic complications of hepatitis B infections include:

- acute viral hepatitis

- fulminant hepatic failure

- chronic active and chronic persistent viral hepatitis

- cirrhosis

- hepatocellular carcinoma.

Chronic carriage of the virus is facilitated by the ability of the hepatitis B virus to integrate into the DNA and to infect hepatocytes that normally express low levels of MHC class I on their cell surface. Both these strategies help the virus to evade the host's defence mechanisms. Damage to the liver usually results from the host's immune response in an attempt to clear the virus (so-called immune pathology).

It is now well recognised that hepatitis B is a risk factor for the development of primary liver cancer (hepatocellular carcinoma). Indeed, after tobacco smoking, hepatitis B is the second most common human carcinogen worldwide.

Hepatitis B is effectively prevented (not treated) by hepatitis B immunisation, which is mandatory for all healthcare professionals who regularly come into contact with blood products. Hepatitis B is treated with serum immunoglobulin and anti-viral agents (interferon-α and lamivudine).

22   D   Establishes persistence though antigenic variation

HIV is an enveloped RNA retrovirus containing two copies of genomic RNA and three viral enzymes (reverse transcriptase, protease and integrase). HIV RNA is transcribed by viral reverse transcriptase into DNA which integrates into the host cell genome. HIV is transmitted by three routes: sexual contact, blood-borne transmission (transfusions or contaminated needles) or vertically from mother to baby (transplacental or via breast milk).

The CD4 antigen on helper T cells is the receptor for the gp120 viral envelope protein, allowing HIV to infect CD4 T cells (helper T cells). The destruction of CD4 cells is central to the pathogenesis of HIV infection. CD4 cells play a pivotal role in the orchestration of both humorally and cell-mediated immune responses. Therefore, by directly infecting and eliminating CD4 cells, HIV leads to a slow and progressive decline in immune function. The end-result is AIDS (acquired immune deficiency syndrome) where the body opens up a whole range of opportunistic infections, the consequences of which are often fatal.

There are several ways in which the HIV evades the host immune system and establishes persistence, eg:

- By directly infecting cells of the immune system, thereby enabling the virus to 'hide' from the immune system.

- By infecting macrophages and dendritic cells in addition to CD4 cells, thereby establishing an important reservoir of infection in lymphoid tissues and forming a site for continued viral replication.

- By directly integrating into the host cell DNA.

- By constantly mutating in a process known as antigenic variation. The generation of new antigenic variants is primarily a function of the high intrinsic error rate present in the reverse transcriptase enzyme (1 in 1000 base-pair error rate). The huge number of variants of HIV in a single infected patient during the course of infection eventually swamps the immune system, leading to its collapse.

23   D   Mutations in the haemagglutinin molecule are responsible for antigenic drift

Viruses can be classified according to:

- particle structure (ie virus family)

- genomic type: RNA or DNA, single stranded or double stranded.

In addition single-stranded RNA viruses can be divided into positive-stranded (coding) and negative-stranded (non-coding) RNA.

Influenza is a member of the *Orthomyxoviridae* family of viruses and has a negative single-stranded RNA genome. The spherical surface of the virus is a lipid bilayer (envelope) containing viral haemagglutinin (HA) and neuramidase (NA), which determine the subtype of the virus. HA mediates the entry of the virus into host cells. NA may be important in the release of viruses from host cells.

Epidemics of influenza occur through mutations, resulting in amino acid substitutions of HA and NA that allow the virus to escape most host antibodies (antigenic drift). Pandemics, which tend to be longer and more widespread then epidemics, may occur when both HA and NA are replaced through recombination of RNA segments with those of animal viruses, making all individuals susceptible to the new influenza virus (antigenic shift). The most notable influenza pandemics occurred in 1918, 1957 and 1968, resulting in millions of deaths worldwide. The virus that caused the last pandemic (H3N2) has been drifting ever since and we have no idea when the next pandemic will occur.

Transmission of influenza occurs by droplet inhalation. The initial symptoms of influenza are a result of direct viral damage and associated inflammatory responses. Life-threatening influenza is often caused by secondary bacterial infection as a result of the destruction of the respiratory epithelium by the influenza virus.

Influenza may be prevented by a vaccine that consists of inactivated preparations of the virus. It provides protection in up to 70% of individuals for about a year. It is recommended for those only at high risk of acquiring the virus. The vaccines in use contain the HA and NA components in relation to the prevalent strain or strains of influenza circulating the previous year. Each year the World Health Organization (WHO) recommends which strains should be included.

24 **B Delayed hypersensitivity reaction against the bacterium**

Mycobacteria stimulate a specific T-cell response of cell-mediated immunity, resulting in granuloma formation. Although this is effective in reducing the infection, the delayed hypersensitivity (type IV) reaction also damages the host tissues. Damage therefore primarily results from the host's immune response in an attempt to clear the body of infection – so-called immune pathology.

The formation of granulomas is the host's attempt to wall off the mycobacteria from the rest of the body, thereby preventing dissemination. When an individual is immunosuppressed (in HIV, for example), dissemination occurs more readily, with disastrous consequences.

The tubercle bacilli can survive within macrophages and this may account for latent infections and reactivation of TB in later life. There is no significant humoral response to mycobacteria. Necrosis does occur in TB, but is usually within the granuloma (caseous necrosis). *M. tuberculosis* causes little or no direct or toxin-mediated damage.

25 **C Typically affects the apical lung in post-primary tuberculosis (TB)**

A third of the world's population are infected with *Mycobacterium tuberculosis*, which is a major cause of death worldwide. It is rapidly increasing in prevalence, in part because of the sharp increase in the number of individuals infected with HIV and the recent emergence of multidrug-resistant TB.

Mycobacteria are obligate, aerobic, rod-shaped, non-spore-forming, non-motile bacilli with a waxy coat that causes them to retain certain stains after being treated with acid and alcohol; they are therefore known as acid–alcohol-fast bacilli (AAFB). Mycobacteria do not readily take up the Gram stain but they would be Gram positive if the Gram stain could penetrate their waxy walls. The Ziehl–Neelsen stain is used instead to visualise the organisms, which stain pink–red.

The pattern of host response depends on whether the infection represents a primary first exposure to the organism (primary TB) or secondary reactivation or reinfection (post-primary or secondary TB). Primary TB is most often subpleural, most often in the periphery of one lung, in the mid-zone. The residuum of the primary infection is a calcified scar in the lung parenchyma (Ghon focus) along with hilar lymph node enlargement; together these are referred to as the Ghon complex. Secondary TB occurs most often at the lung apex (Assman lesion) of one or both lungs, which may cavitate and heal by dense fibrosis. The apex of the lung is more highly oxygenated, allowing the aerobic mycobacteria to multiply more rapidly. Involvement of extrapulmonary sites (eg the kidney, meninges, bone) is not uncommon.

M. tuberculosis is resistant to penicillin and requires multimodal antibiotic therapy (which may be remembered by RIPE – see below) to prevent the emergence of resistance:

- rifampicin (main side effect: liver toxicity)
- isoniazid (main side effect: peripheral neuropathy)
- pyrazinamide (main side effect: liver toxicity)
- ethambutol (main side effect: optic neuropathy with visual disturbances).

Several months of combination treatment are required to treat *M. tuberculosis*. Pyridoxine (vitamin B_6) should be given with isoniazid to prevent isoniazid neuropathy.

M. tuberculosis can be prevented by immunisation with BCG (Bacille Calmette–Guérin), a vaccine made from non-virulent tubercle bacilli. However, the protective efficacy of the vaccine is variable, ranging from 0 to 80% depending on the part of the world in which it is administered.

26   C   Results from the secretion of exotoxin

All members of the clostridia group of organisms have the following properties:

- all Gram-positive bacilli
- all obligate anaerobes
- all spore forming
- all saprophytic (ie live in the soil)
- all motile (but non-invasive)
- exotoxin producing.

Clostridia are responsible for causing several diseases in humans: *Clostridium tetani* (tetanus), *C. botulinum* (botulism), *C. perfringens*, formerly known as *C. welchii* (gas gangrene and food poisoning), and *C. difficile* (pseudomembranous colitis).

Tetanus is typically a disease of soldiers, farmers or gardeners. It is a result of deep penetrating wounds caused by objects contaminated with soil, which introduces spores into the tissue. As soon as the wound becomes anaerobic, the tetanus spores germinate to produce vegetative cells, which then multiply and release a potent neurotoxin called tetanospasmin. Only the tiniest quantities of exotoxin are needed for the disease to develop. The bacteria producing the exotoxin are entirely non-invasive and lack all other virulence factors apart from the capacity to produce toxin.

The exotoxin binds to local nerve endings, travels up the axon to the spinal cord, traverses a synaptic junction and finally gains entry to the cytoplasm of inhibitory neurons. Within these cells the toxin exerts a highly specific proteolytic activity on one of the proteins (synaptobrevin) present in the vesicles, which is responsible for the normal trafficking of inhibitory neurotransmitter to the synaptic junction. As a result the inhibitory neuron cannot transmit its impulse and there is unopposed stimulation of skeletal muscles by motor neurons. Death is normally a result of muscular spasm (spastic paralysis) extending to involve the muscles of the chest so that the patient is unable to breathe.

As in other diseases caused entirely by an exotoxin, tetanus can be treated by passive immunisation with antitoxin, and prevented by immunisation with toxoid. However, antitoxin cannot neutralise any toxin that has already entered neurons. Antibiotics are of limited value against anaerobic bacteria such as clostridia because they cannot penetrate the necrotic infected area in sufficient concentrations to be effective; surgical débridement of wounds is far superior.

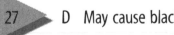

27   D   May cause blackwater fever

Malaria is a worldwide infection that affects 500 million and kills 3 million people (mostly children) every year; it is therefore the major parasitic cause of death and is the most deadly vector-borne disease in the world. Malaria is caused by protozoan parasites of the genus *Plasmodium*. There are four main species that infect humans: *Plasmodium falciparum, P. vivax, P. malariae* and *P. ovale.*

Of these *P. falciparum* is the most virulent, widespread and drug resistant, and causes the most morbidity and mortality through its ability to cause cerebral malaria, severe anaemia, hypoglycaemia, lactic acidosis, renal failure, pulmonary oedema and shock ('algid malaria'). Blackwater fever is characterised by intravascular haemolysis, haemoglobinuria and kidney failure.

P. falciparum is the most pathogenic strain for two principal reasons:

1. *P. falciparum* can develop in red cells of all ages; the other less pathogenic species are limited to growing in subpopulations of cells – either very young or very mature cells. *P. falciparum* can therefore cause higher levels of parasitaemia.

2. The distinctive behaviour of *P. falciparum*-infected red cells – namely cytoadherence to vascular endothelium and sequestration, which minimises removal of infected erythrocytes by the spleen.

Plasmodia are transmitted to humans by more than a dozen species of female anopheles mosquitoes, which require a blood meal before they can breed (the aedes mosquito acts as a vector for yellow fever and dengue fever, not malaria). The male mosquitoes feed harmlessly on plant sap. The anopheles mosquito vector is also the definitive host in which sexual reproduction occurs, so fertilisation occurs in the insect, not in the human!

Malaria is treated with supportive management and chemotherapy. Preventive strategies include chemoprophylaxis (which is by no means 100% effective!), vector control (such as insecticides) and bite prevention (insect repellents, mosquito nets, covering up exposed areas especially at dawn and dusk). Unfortunately, at present there is no effective immunisation for the prevention of malaria. The quest to develop a malaria vaccine is currently an active area of research.

B   Parasites may remain dormant in the liver as
hypnozoites

The malaria parasite has a complex life cycle. In their definitive
host (the mosquito), the parasites undergo a cycle of sexual and
asexual development. In their intermediate host (the human),
they undergo two cycles of asexual development (in the liver
and red blood cells). In addition there are alternating and
extracellular stages.

The genetic recombination allowed by the sexual stage is one
element in the remarkable antigenic diversity seen within
malaria parasite populations that enables it to evade the immune
response. The malaria life cycle is easiest to understand if it is
broken down into three stages:

1. The intermediate host (humans): hepatic stage. Human
    infection begins when sporozoites are introduced into an
    individual's bloodstream as an infected mosquito takes a
    blood meal. Within 30 min, they disappear from the blood as
    they infect hepatocytes. Here they undergo the first round of
    asexual reproduction (exoerythrocytic shizogeny) and
    develop into exoerythrocytic schizonts. These
    exoerythrocytic schizonts may contain many thousands of
    merozoites. On invasion of the hepatocyte by *P. vivax* and *P.
    ovale*, the development of the schizont is retarded, and a
    'dormant' stage of the parasite, the hypnozoite, is formed.
    This is responsible for disease relapse months to years after
    supposed chemotherapeutic cure and clearance of
    bloodstream forms of the parasite.

2. The intermediate host (humans): erythrocytic stage. The
    released merozoites infect red cells where they undergo
    another round of asexual reproduction (erythocytic
    schizogeny) changing from merozoite to trophozoite (feeding
    stage) to schizont. Eventually the cell ruptures and releases

new merozoites (usually between 8 and 32), which go on to infect more red cells. Generally the parasite's life cycle stages are highly synchronised, such that at any one time all the parasites are at the trophozoite stage or at the schizont stage. Fever in malaria is either tertian (every 48 hours in *P. falciparum, P. vivax* and *P. ovale*) or quartan (every 72 hours in *P. malariae*) and is the result of the synchronised release of merozoites from red cells. Malignant tertian fever is caused by *P. falciparum*. In addition, on infection of new blood cells, instead of forming trophozoites the parasites may grow into the immature gametocytes. These are not released from the red cell until taken up by a feeding mosquito.

3. The determinate host (mosquito). The female anopheles mosquitoes ingest blood as part of their lifecycle. Here the normal asexually dividing bloodstream forms die, but the gametocytes are stimulated to mature to microgametes (male) and macrogametes (female). Fertilisation occurs in the mosquito midgut, resulting in the formation of a zygote. This then goes on to produce a worm-like form, the ookinete, which penetrates the midgut wall of the mosquito, forming an oocyst located between the epithelium and the basement membrane. Note that the zygote is the sole diploid stage of malaria parasites; the only meiosis event during this life cycle occurs within a few hours of zygote formation. Within the oocyst a cycle of asexual reproduction (sporogeny) takes place, with the formation of numerous sporozoites. When mature, the oocyst bursts open, releasing these sporozoites, which then migrate to the insect's salivary glands. From here they may enter the bloodstream of a new host, thus completing the parasite's life cycle.

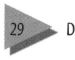

29 ▶ D Disease results from the immune response to schistosome eggs

Parasitic infections may be caused by protozoa or metazoa. Parasitic protozoa (eg *Plasmodium falciparum*) are single-celled nucleate organisms that possess all the processes necessary for reproduction. Metazoan are multicellular organisms. Examples of infective metazoa include helminths (parasitic worms), which can be subdivided into three classes: nematodes (roundworms), cestodes (flatworms) and trematodes (flukes).

Schistosomiasis is the most important helminth disease infecting 200 million people worldwide. Three major species of schistosome parasite can infect humans: *Schistosoma mansoni, S. japonicum* and *S. haematobium*. All are trematodes (flukes).

The life cycle of the flatworms that cause human schistosomiasis involves a sexual stage in the human (the definitive host) and an asexual stage in the fresh water snail host, which acts as a vector or intermediate host. Schistosome eggs excreted in the faeces or urine hatch out in fresh water and release miracidia that invade snails; free-swimming cercaria are released from the snail and invade human skin, losing their tails and becoming known as schistosomulae. The larvae migrate through the bloodstream via the lungs and liver to the veins of the bladder (*S. haematobium*) or bowel (*S. mansoni, S. japonicum*) where they develop into adult males and females. The adults lay eggs, which are excreted by the host, thus completing the cycle.

The pathophysiology of schistosomiasis is mainly caused by the immune response against the schistosome eggs. In the liver this may result in granuloma formation, extensive fibrosis (pipe-stem portal fibrosis) and portal hypertension (hepatosplenic schistosomiasis). *S. haematobium* is responsible for urinary schistosomiasis, where granulomatous inflammation and fibrosis in the bladder may result in haematuria, obstructive uropathy

ANSWERS

Medical microbiology – Answers

and squamous cell carcinoma of the bladder. Schistosomiasis is treated with praziquantel, which removes the flukes, but in advanced cases the pathology is irreversible. Intense inflammatory reactions are provoked when the worms killed by treatment are carried back into the liver.

30 ▶ E Are responsible for causing kuru in humans

Prions are novel, infectious agents composed of protein only. They differ from all known pathogens. They lack nucleic acid and cannot be considered micro-organisms. They are highly resistant to decontamination methods such as standard autoclaving (heat), disinfectants (chemicals) and ionising radiation.

If abnormal prion protein is inoculated into a normal host, conformational changes are induced in the normal host prions, resulting in their conversion to abnormal host prions. These then induce further conformational changes in remaining normal host prions. Thus, the original inoculated protein is able to catalyse a chain reaction in which host proteins become conformationally abnormal. This is not accompanied by inflammation, immune reaction or cytokine release.

Well-known prion diseases include kuru, scrapie, bovine spongiform encephalopathy (BSE) and Creutzfeldt–Jakob disease (CJD). Kuru is probably one of the most fascinating stories to have emerged from any epidemiological investigation. It occurred in villages occupied by the Fore tribes in the highlands of New Guinea who practised ritual cannibalism as a rite of mourning for their dead. The first cases occurred in the 1950s and involved progressive loss of voluntary control, followed by death within a year of the onset of symptoms. Interestingly, kuru occurred only in individuals who participated in cannibalistic feasts. Such cannibalism was believed to be responsible for the transmission of prions in kuru.

There is still much work to be done in determining the exact modes of transmission of prions and in enhancing our understanding of their molecular biology. In addition the exact interrelations between the different prion-related diseases (eg BSE and new variant CJD) needs to be clarified.

Cancer biology
Answers

31   **D   Anaplasia is almost a complete lack of differentiation**

There are certain definitions about tumours that need to be remembered and understood:

- Tumour simply means 'swelling'. It can be benign or malignant.

- Neoplasm simply means a 'new growth'. It is synonymous with tumour and can be benign or malignant. Malignant neoplasms can be primary or secondary. The latter are also known as metastases.

- Hypertrophy is an increase in tissue growth through an increase in cell size.

- Hyperplasia is an increase in tissue growth through an increase in cell number.

- Metaplasia is an adaptive response, resulting in the replacement of one differentiated cell type by another.

- Dysplasia is best remembered because it literally means 'disordered growth'. It is the disordered development of cells resulting in an alteration in their size, shape and organisation.

- Carcinoma in situ is an epithelial tumour with features of malignancy, but it has not invaded through the basement membrane.

- Carcinoma is a malignant tumour of epithelial derivation. By definition, as it is malignant, the basement membrane has been breached.

- Anaplasia is the almost complete lack of differentiation (ie poorly differentiated).

A more formal definition of a neoplasm is 'an abnormal mass of tissue, the growth of which exceeds and is uncoordinated with that of the normal tissues, and persists in the same excessive manner after cessation of the stimuli that evoked the change'. The last part of this definition is to distinguish a true neoplasm from the endometrial growth that normally accompanies the menstrual cycle: endometrial tissue is normally responsive to sex hormones and regresses on their cessation; a true neoplasm would persist.

32   E   Liposarcoma is a malignant tumour of adipose tissue

In general, benign tumours are designated by attaching the suffix -oma to the cell of origin. Thus an adenoma is a benign tumour of glandular epithelial cells. However, there are exceptions to this rule, eg a lymphoma is a malignant lymphoreticular tumour.

Malignant tumours arising from connective tissue are called sarcomas. Thus a liposarcoma is a malignant tumour of adipose tissue, a leiomyosarcoma is a malignant tumour of smooth muscle and a rhabdomyosarcoma is a malignant tumour of skeletal muscle. Malignant tumours of epithelial origin are called carcinomas. Thus, an adenocarcinoma is a malignant neoplasm of glandular epithelium and squamous cell carcinomas are malignant neoplasms arising from squamous epithelium.

C Metaplasia in the bronchus involves a change from columnar to stratified squamous epithelium

Metaplasia is the reversible change of one fully differentiated cell type into another fully differentiated cell type, in response to injury. It often represents an adaptive response to environmental stress. Squamous metaplasia is by far the most common. Its significance lies in the fact that it can become dysplastic if the agent that caused the metaplasia persists and is capable of inducing dysplasia.

Important sites of metaplasia:

- The lower end of the oesophagus in response to acid reflux (Barrett's oesophagus). The normal stratified squamous epithelium is replaced by gastric-type columnar epithelium, which is able to produce mucus and protect the epithelium from acid reflux.

- In the bronchi, where the normal respiratory (ciliated columnar) epithelium is replaced by stratified squamous epithelium under the influence of chronic irritation by cigarette smoke (squamous metaplasia).

- Transformation zone of the cervix: in response to environmental changes during the reproductive cycle and to human papilloma virus, the normal columnar endocervical epithelium is replaced by stratified squamous epithelium.

- Squamous metaplasia of the bladder in response to chronic inflammation, infection and irritation (schistosomiasis, calculi, etc).

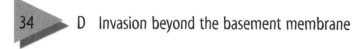

34 ▶ D Invasion beyond the basement membrane

The defining and most reliable characteristic differentiating a benign from a malignant tumour is the ability of the latter to invade through the basement membrane into the surrounding tissues and metastasise to distant sites.

Both benign and malignant tumours increase in size with time. However, malignant tumours tend to grow more rapidly and aggressively than benign tumours. The result is that malignant tumours tend to outstrip their blood supply, leading to necrosis. Haemorrhage occurs as a result of the fragile new vasculature that forms in an attempt to increase blood supply to the tumour.

Chromosomal abnormalities do not define a tumour as malignant because this may be a feature of both benign and malignant tumours. The presence of a pseudo-capsule is typically a feature of benign lesions and results from the neoplasm expanding symmetrically and compressing the surrounding stroma. Such encapsulation tends to contain the benign neoplasm as a discrete, readily palpable and easily movable mass, which can be surgically enucleated because there is a well-defined cleavage plane around the tumour.

In general, benign tumours are well differentiated, meaning that the tumour cells resemble the normal mature cells of the tissue of origin of the neoplasm and display well-ordered maturation. Malignant tumours, in contrast, range from well differentiated to undifferentiated or poorly differentiated. Malignant tumours composed of undifferentiated cells are said to be anaplastic.

ANSWERS

MCQs in Applied Basic Sciences for Medical Students: Volume 2

Both cytology and histology involve the study of cells at the microscopic level. Cytology studies individual cells and cell morphology. Histology studies cells within the context of tissues and provides information about tissue architecture. Only histology can provide definitive diagnosis of invasion.

The cytological features of malignancy include:

- increased nuclear:cytoplasmic ratio
- hyperchromatism (darkly staining nuclei resulting from increased amounts of DNA)
- prominent nucleoli
- variability in cellular and nuclear size and shape (cellular and nuclear pleomorphism)
- high mitotic index (increased mitotic rate)
- abnormal mitotic figures
- lack of differentiation (anaplasia).

The histological features of malignancy include all of the above, plus:

- loss of normal tissue architecture
- infiltrative borders, with a disordered growth pattern
- invasion beyond the basement membrane
- lymphovascular involvement
- excessive necrosis and haemorrhage
- loss of cell–cell cohesion, resulting in shedding

Pyknosis, karyorrhexis and karyolysis are cytological features of cell death (necrosis and apoptosis), rather than malignancy.

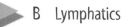

36 ▶ B Lymphatics

Metastasis is the seeding of tumour cells to sites distant and detached from the primary tumour. This is different to invasion, which is spread in continuity.

As a general rule, carcinomas (malignant tumours of epithelial origin) most often metastasise via the lymph; sarcomas (malignant tumours of connective tissue origin) most often metastasise via the bloodstream.

Thus, breast carcinomas often spread to local lymph nodes (axillary and internal mammary), whereas osteosarcomas typically spread via the bloodstream, forming cannon-ball metastases in the lungs. However, this rule is slightly misleading because ultimately there are numerous interconnections between the vascular and lymphatic systems. In addition, every rule has exceptions (eg follicular carcinoma of the thyroid spreads by the haematogenous route).

Neoplasms, in general, may metastasise by several routes:

- local invasion (direct spread)
- via the bloodstream (haematogenous route)
- via the lymphatics
- transcoelomic spread (eg across the peritoneal or pleural cavities)
- via the cerebrospinal fluid (CSF) (for CNS tumours)
- perineural spread (eg adenoid cystic carcinoma of the parotid)
- implantation/accidental seeding during surgery – iatrogenic

ANSWERS

MCQs in Applied Basic Sciences for Medical Students: Volume 2

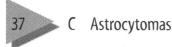

37   C   Astrocytomas

It is estimated that 50% of bronchial carcinomas have metastasised by the time of clinical presentation.

Breast carcinoma metastasises readily to sites such as the lung, bone and brain. Melanoma is an aggressive tumour that can metastasise to virtually any site within the body. It therefore carries an extremely poor prognosis. Renal cell carcinomas characteristically invade the renal veins and extend into the inferior vena cava (sometimes reaching as far as the right atrium), so that blood-borne metastases are common, especially to the lungs, liver and bone.

Astrocytomas (and even the poorly differentiated form, glioblastoma multiforme), rarely metastasise to sites outside the CNS because they are contained by the blood–brain barrier. They usually metastasise outside the CNS only if there is a breach in the blood–brain barrier or an artificial connection (such as a ventriculoperitoneal shunt) connecting the CNS with another part of the body.

38   C   Have a peak incidence in those aged less than 50

Carcinomas are much more common than sarcomas. The former are malignant neoplasms derived from epithelium, whereas the latter are malignant neoplasms derived from connective tissue. Sarcomas have a peak incidence in those younger than 50.

The preferred route of metastasis for sarcomas is via the bloodstream; this contrasts with carcinomas, which usually metastasise via the lymphatics. Understandably the liver and lungs are most frequently involved secondarily in such haematogenous dissemination because all portal drainage flows to the liver and all caval blood flows to the lungs.

No in situ phase has been identified for sarcomas, unlike in carcinomas where there is often an in situ phase. As a result sarcomas generally carry a poor prognosis.

39 ▶ B Tumour growth obeys gompertzian kinetics

If we consider the growth of a tumour, one cell divides to form two cells; these divide to form four cells, and so on. Assuming no cell loss tumours will grow, doubling in cell number every few days (a typical cell cycle in a mammalian cell lasts about 24 hours).

Cells continue to multiply because there is loss of the normal regulatory mechanisms that restrict tissue growth (such as contact inhibition). It is unusual for a tumour to become clinically obvious until there are about 10^9 cells (30 divisions), or 1 gram of tumour cells (corresponding to a tumour diameter of about 1 cm).

However, as the tumour continues to grow it begins to outstrip its own blood supply so that an increasing number of cells are lost by apoptosis. In addition as the tumour expands more and more cells are shed through exfoliation, hypoxia, non-viability, metastasis and host defences.

The result of this is twofold: first, the rate of tumour growth begins to slow down from the initial exponential pattern of growth, and the tumour growth curve therefore tends to assume a sigmoidal shape (gompertzian kinetics); second, it means that the growth fraction (the proportion of cells within the tumour population that is in the proliferative pool) of smaller tumours is greater than that of larger tumours.

As tumours continue to grow, cells leave the replicative pool in ever-increasing numbers, as a result of shedding or lack of nutrients, by differentiating and reversion to the resting phase of the cell cycle, G_0. Thus, by the time the tumour is clinically detectable, most cells are not in the replicative pool (and therefore are relatively resistant to the effects of chemoradiotherapy). The growth fraction is usually 4–80%, with an average of less than 20%. Even in some rapidly growing tumours, the growth fraction is only about 20%. Indeed, some normal tissues, such as bone marrow and alimentary mucosa, have larger growth fractions and shorter mitotic cycle times than many cancers, even cancers of those tissues. Ultimately, the progressive growth of tumours and the rate at which they grow are determined by the excess of cell production over cell loss.

It is very important to recognise that the clinical phase of a tumour, which is the time from it becoming clinically apparent until it causes the death of the patient (assuming no treatment), is short in comparison to the pre-clinical phase. Thus, by the time a solid tumour has been detected, it has already completed a major portion of its lifecycle. During the long pre-clinical phase there is time for invasion and metastasis to occur. In addition there is time for cell heterogeneity to develop within the tumour. This means that over and above the initial mutations, further genetic events occur in subpopulations of the tumour, leading to variation and the outgrowth of subpopulations with different patterns of differentiation and properties (a form of darwinian evolution).

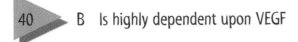

40   B   Is highly dependent upon VEGF

As soon as tumours grow to more than about 1–2 mm³ they require the development of new blood vessels to sustain them – a process called angiogenesis (not to be confused with apoptosis which is programmed cell death).

This is because the zone of 1–2 mm represents the maximal distance across which oxygen and nutrients can diffuse from blood vessels. Beyond 1–2 mm the tumour fails to enlarge without blood vascularisation because hypoxia induces apoptosis by activation of *p53*. Neovascularisation has a dual effect on tumour growth: perfusion supplies nutrients and oxygen to the growing tumour and newly formed endothelial cells stimulate the growth of adjacent tumour cells through the secretion of cytokines.

Tumour cells elaborate factors called angiogenic factors that induce new blood vessel formation. Of the dozen or so tumour-associated angiogenic factors that have been discovered so far, the two most important are vascular endothelial growth factor (VEGF) and basic fibroblast growth factor (bFGF). Much attention has focused on the use of angiogenesis inhibitors to cure cancer because angiogenesis is critical for the growth and metastasis of tumours. Whether this theoretical benefit translates into clinical practice is another matter and clinical trials are currently in progress.

Angiogenesis is also a hallmark of granulation tissue. It plays an important physiological role in wound healing by assisting in the delivery of oxygen and nutrients to healing tissue, where it is required for growth and repair. Granulation tissue produces a rich 'cytokine soup', including secretion of VEGF and bFGF, which stimulate angiogenesis.

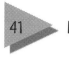

41 **D** Hepatocellular carcinoma and polyvinyl chloride
exposure

A carcinogen is a substance, form of energy or organism capable
of inducing a cancer. The following carcinogens have been
strongly associated with the workplace:

- scrotal cancer (Pott's cancer) in chimney sweeps

- mesotheliomas in people exposed to asbestos (workers in
  the building industry, ship construction and demolition)

- transitional cell carcinoma of the bladder in rubber and
  dye workers, caused by exposure to β-naphthylamine

- angiosarcomas in workers exposed to polyvinyl chloride

- skin carcinoma in workers exposed to ultraviolet radiation
  (principally outdoor occupations, eg farmers).

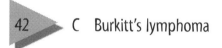

42 **C** Burkitt's lymphoma

Oncogenic micro-organisms are micro-organisms that are
capable of producing tumours. Most are viral. However,
Helicobacter pylori is a good example of a bacterium that has
been associated with gastric carcinoma and gastric lymphoma,
and *Schistosoma haematobium* is a good example of a parasitic
infection that is capable of producing squamous cell carcinoma
of the bladder.

Viruses are obligate intracellular parasites that rely on the host
cell's replicative machinery to reproduce themselves. Oncogenic
viruses have therefore evolved to induce host cell replication
by activating genes for cell growth. This confers a survival

advantage upon the virus. However, it is when proliferation becomes unco-ordinated and excessive that carcinoma results.

EBV (DNA) has been implicated in the pathogenesis of three human cancers:

1. Burkitt's lymphoma
2. Nasopharyngeal carcinoma
3. Hodgkin's disease.

Other well-described oncogenic viruses, besides EBV, include:

RNA oncogenic viruses:

- Human T-cell leukaemia virus (HTLV-1) → human T-cell leukaemia
- Hepatitis C virus → hepatocellular carcinoma.

DNA oncogenic viruses:

- Hepatitis B virus (HBV) → hepatocellular carcinoma
- Human herpes virus type 8 (HHV-8) → Kaposi's sarcoma (in individuals who are HIV positive)
- Human papilloma virus (HPV) → cervical carcinoma; anal carcinoma.

There are several mechanisms by which viruses can induce malignancy:

- Directly, by becoming integrated into a cell's genome and by activation of cellular oncogenes
- Indirectly, through processes (eg chronic inflammation) that predispose to malignancy. The mitotically active tissue presumably provides a fertile soil for mutations
- By the production of proteins that inactivate tumour-suppressor proteins, such as p53.

A They behave in dominant fashion

Cancer is a genetic disease. Oncogenes are growth-promoting genes that are expressed in normal cells (the correct name for its normal precursor is proto-oncogene). They encode for oncoproteins (growth factors, growth receptor molecules, signal transducing molecules, nuclear transcription factors, regulators of the cell cycle) that positively regulate growth, and are involved in the growth and differentiation of normal cells.

Transcription of oncogenes is tightly regulated in normal cells.

Overexpression of oncoproteins, or mutations of oncogenes resulting in the inappropriate activation of oncoproteins, leads to abnormal cell growth and survival (ie tumorigenesis). Mutations in oncogenes that result in tumours are generally gain-of-function mutations and thus oncogenes behave in a dominant manner to promote cell transformation, ie only one copy of the defective gene is sufficient to cause cancer.

Proto-oncogenes are converted into oncogenes through a variety of different mechanisms that include:

- point mutations
- chromosomal rearrangements
- gene amplification
- incorporation of a new promoter (by viruses)
- incorporation of enhancer sequences (by viruses).

The last two mechanisms are also referred to as insertional mutagenesis.

BRCA-1 is a tumour-suppressor gene that accounts for a small proportion of breast cancers.

ANSWERS

Cancer biology – Answers

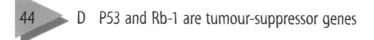

44 D P53 and Rb-1 are tumour-suppressor genes

Tumour-suppressor genes encode proteins that negatively regulate cell proliferation and thus suppress tumour growth. Both *p53* and *Rb-1* are good examples located on chromosomes 17 and 13, respectively. Normal *p53* is the so-called 'guardian of the genome' and triggers apoptosis and cell cycle arrest in genetically damaged cells (ie it is pro-apoptotic).

Mutations in *p53* therefore result in the propagation of genetically damaged cells and tumorigenesis. Indeed, about 50% of human tumours contain mutations in *p53*, and *p53*-related cancers are more aggressive and have a poorer prognosis.

In contrast to oncogenes, tumours caused by tumour-suppressor genes are generally the result of mutations causing a loss of function of the gene product; neoplastic growth resulting from the loss of the protective role of tumour-suppressor genes. Loss of tumour-suppressor function usually requires the inactivation of both alleles of the gene, so that all the protective effect of tumour-suppressor genes is lost, ie they are generally deemed to behave in a recessive manner.

Cellular proliferation is therefore tightly regulated by two sets of opposing functioning genes: the growth-promoting genes (proto-oncogenes) and the negative cell cycle regulators (tumour-suppressor genes). Abnormal activation of proto-oncogenes and/or loss of function of tumour-suppressor genes leads to the transformation of a normal cell into a cancer cell.

Retinoblastoma is a fascinating condition and important to know about. Much is known about retinoblastoma because the gene responsible for the condition was the first tumour-suppressor gene to be discovered.

In addition, study of the tumour has provided us with valuable information on how tumour-suppressor genes function. Retinoblastoma is caused by a mutation in *Rb-1* (a tumour-suppressor gene) on the long arm of chromosome 13. About 60% of cases are sporadic and 40% inherited, being transmitted as an autosomal dominant trait. Although inherited in this fashion, cancer results only when both copies of the normal gene are lost. This apparent paradox is explained by Knudson's two-hit hypothesis.

Knudson suggested that, in inherited cases, one genetic change (first hit) is inherited from an affected parent (ie the condition is inherited in an autosomal dominant manner) and is therefore present in all somatic cells of the body, whereas the second mutation (second hit) occurs after birth through some form of somatic mutation in one of the many retinal cells (which already carry the first mutation). In other words, loss of heterozygosity of the normal *Rb* gene results in cancer.

The mutation rate for the gene is thought to be 1:10 000 000, about the same as the number of divisions that are needed to form the adult retina; thus the chance of a somatic mutation occurring in an individual with only one functioning gene is very high. In sporadic cases, however, both mutations (hits) occur somatically within a single retinal cell. Patients with familial forms of retinoblastomas are at increased risk of developing extraretinal cancers (such as osteosarcomas) because the newborn child carries an inherited mutant *Rb* allele in all somatic cells of the body.

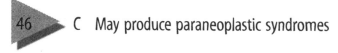

Currently lung cancer is the most common cause of death from cancer in both men and women. It is estimated that some 50% of bronchial carcinomas have metastasised by the time of clinical presentation. Lung carcinoma is most commonly due to squamous cell carcinoma, which is usually caused by squamous cell metaplasia as a result of smoking.

Tobacco smoking is believed to account for 80–90% of cases of lung carcinoma; the remainder are associated with radon gas and asbestos exposure.

The pathological effects of any tumour may be local or distant; distant effects may be metastatic or non-metastatic (paraneoplastic). Applying this to lung carcinoma we have the following effects.

Local effects:

- Pulmonary involvement – cough (infection distal to airway blocked by tumour as a result of disruption of the mucociliary escalator), haemoptysis (ulceration/necrosis of tumour), breathlessness (local extension of tumour), chest pain (involvement of pleura and/or chest wall), wheeze (narrowing of airways).

- Local invasion: hoarseness (recurrent laryngeal nerve infiltration), Horner syndrome (infiltration of the ipsilateral sympathetic chain), wasting of the intrinsic hand muscles (brachial plexus infiltration), diaphragmatic paralysis (phrenic nerve invasion), pleural effusions (tumour spread into pleura), pericarditis (pericardial involvement), superior vena cava obstruction (direct compression by tumour).

Distant effects:

- Metastatic: pathological fractures (bone metastases), neurological symptoms (brain metastases), hepatomegaly or jaundice (liver metastases).

- Non-metastatic (paraneoplastic) effects: ectopic hormone production (ADH, ACTH, PTHrP, serotonin, etc), common generalised symptoms (weight loss, anorexia, lassitude) from the acute phase response (IL-1, IL-6, TNF-α).

Paraneoplastic syndromes are symptoms and signs associated with a malignant tumour that is not the result of direct local effects of the tumour or the development of metastases.

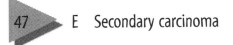

47   E   Secondary carcinoma

Tumours or neoplasms may be benign or malignant. Malignant tumours may be primary or secondary. The most common intracerebral neoplasms are secondaries, accounting for about 50% of all intracerebral tumours. The five most common primary sites are the lung, breast, skin (melanoma), kidney and gastrointestinal tract.

Ninety per cent of normal brain tissue is composed of glial (supporting) cells, whereas the remaining 10% are composed of neurons, ie there are about 10 times as many glia as there are neurons in normal brain parenchyma. Primary intracerebral neoplasms therefore predominantly arise from the glial cells, rather than the neurons. Astrocytoma is the most common type of glioma. Meningiomas originate from the arachnoid granulations and press into the brain tissue from outside.

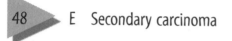
Tumours or neoplasms may be benign or malignant. Malignant tumours may be primary or secondary. Secondary bone tumours (ie metastases) are the most common malignant tumour of bone, occurring in 70% of patients with disseminated malignant disease.

They are more common than all the primary malignant tumours put together. After the liver and lung, the bone is the third most common site for metastatic spread. The most common primary malignant tumour of bone is the osteosarcoma.

The six most common tumours that spread to bone are:

- multiple myeloma
- breast
- bronchus (lung)
- prostate
- kidney
- thyroid (follicular subtype).

Secondary bone tumours may be associated with an osteolytic (bone-dissolving) or osteoblastic (bone-forming) reaction within the bone. Interestingly, both prostate and breast carcinomas have a propensity to form osteoblastic lesions within the bone. The direct effect of metastatic tumours on the bone is one explanation for the hypercalcaemia that is commonly seen in malignancy. Other factors, however, also seem to play a role, such as the release of parathyroid hormone-related protein (PTHrP) by tumour cells.

Principles of pathology
Answers

49 ▶ **D** May be seen in histological section

Apoptosis (from the Greek meaning 'to fall off' as in the leaves of a tree) is programmed cell death. It acts to eliminate unwanted cells or damaged cells with abnormal DNA. It involves the death of individual cells, rather than of large groups of adjacent cells (which is usually the case in necrosis).

Apoptosis is usually unaccompanied by inflammation (inflammation is evident in necrosis). A key feature of apoptosis is that cells can be eliminated with minimal disruption to adjacent cells.

Apoptosis may be physiological (as a normal part of growth and development), as well as pathological, where balance of the production of new cells enables a stable cell population. A good example of physiological apoptosis is the shaping of the hands in embryogenesis. Under normal conditions, apoptosis is precisely regulated by pro-apoptotic (*p53*, *c-myc*, *Bax*, *Bad*) and anti-apoptotic (*Bcl-2*, *Bcl-XL*) factors. Alteration in the fine balance of pro-apoptotic and anti-apoptotic factors may result in neoplasia (eg loss of *p53* is found in many tumours).

Apoptosis is clearly visible in histological sections; apoptotic cells are seen as rounded membrane-bound bodies ('apoptotic bodies'). These bodies are eventually phagocytosed and digested by adjacent cells so that no clump of cellular debris is left permanently behind. The key differences between necrosis and apoptosis are summarised below:

Apoptosis	Necrosis
Energy dependent (active process)	Energy independent
Internally programmed or 'suicide'	Response to external injury
Affects single cells	Affects groups of cells
No accompanying inflammation	Accompanied by inflammation
Physiological or pathological	Always pathological
Plasma membrane remains intact	Loss of plasma membrane integrity
Cell shrinkage, fragmentation and formation of apoptotic bodies	Cell swelling and lysis

D Inflammation is intimately connected with the clotting system

Acute inflammation is a stereotyped, non-specific response to tissue injury. It occurs in response to a variety of different tissue insults (both exogenous or endogenous) and not just from infection, eg it occurs after ischaemia (hypoxic injury), physical trauma or in response to noxious chemicals, such as insect bites.

Inflammation is fundamentally a protective response, the ultimate goal of which is to rid the organism of both the initial cause of cell injury (eg microbes, toxins) and the consequences of such injury (eg necrotic tissues). In some situations, however, inflammation may be harmful to the host (a good example is meningitis).

The four cardinal features of acute inflammation are redness (*rubor*), swelling (*tumour*), heat (*calor*) and pain (*dolor*). Some also add a fifth, such as loss of function (*functio laesa*) or increased secretion (*fluor*). Acute inflammation is part of the innate immune response occurring before the development of any adaptive immune response that may later occur. In this way acute inflammation acts as a 'danger signal' augmenting the adaptive immune response. The inflammatory response is immediate, but non-specific, whereas the adaptive immune response is slower to develop but highly specific, and it acquires memory.

Acute inflammation is initiated by a variety of chemical mediators, all of which interact in a synergistic manner to produce inflammation. These include bacterially derived products, histamine, serotonin, arachidonic acid metabolites, cytokines, and members of the complement, kinin, clotting and fibrinolytic systems. The clotting system and inflammation are intimately connected. Therefore, bleeding at the site of injury can initiate acute inflammation.

ANSWERS

Principles of pathology – Answers

There are three main phases of acute inflammation:

1. Widespread vasodilatation (hyperaemia)

2. Increased vascular permeability

3. Leukocyte extravasation and phagocytosis.

The predominant cell type in acute inflammation is the neutrophil (the macrophage predominates in chronic inflammation). Acute inflammation is of relatively short duration, lasting for minutes, several hours or a few days. If it persists for longer, it is generally regarded as chronic inflammation.

51 D Amyloidosis

The four possible outcomes of acute inflammation are:

1. Resolution (with the complete restoration of normal tissue architecture and function)

2. Abscess formation (an abscess is a localised collection of pus surrounded by granulation tissue; pus is a collection of neutrophils in association with dead and dying organisms)

3. Progression to chronic inflammation

4. Death (a good example being meningitis).

Amyloidosis follows chronic inflammation, rather than acute inflammation.

B Usually heals by organisation and repair

Chronic inflammation is inflammation of prolonged duration (weeks or months) in which active inflammation, tissue destruction and attempts at repair occur simultaneously. It may follow acute inflammation (secondary chronic inflammation), or occur *de novo* in the absence of a preceding acute inflammatory phase (primary chronic inflammation).

Chronic inflammation arises in situations where the injurious stimulus persists, as when:

- the injurious agent is endogenous (eg acid in stomach and peptic ulceration)
- the injurious agent is non-degradable (eg dust particles in pneumoconiosis)
- the injurious agent evades host defence mechanisms (eg many intracellular organisms such as TB)
- the host attacks components of self (eg autoimmunity)
- host resistance (immunity) is suppressed (eg malnutrition, HIV).

Neutrophils are a feature of acute, rather than chronic, inflammation. Chronic inflammation is characterised by more extensive tissue destruction than acute inflammation as a result of the lengthy nature of the process and the greater lysosomal rupture with the release of numerous lytic enzymes. The destroyed tissue is replaced by granulation tissue. Healing occurs by organisation and repair (with fibrosis leaving a scar), rather than through resolution (which is typical of acute inflammation).

The pathological consequences of chronic inflammation include:

- tissue destruction and scarring

- development of cancer – the mitotically active tissue provides a fertile ground for the accumulation of mutations

- amyloidosis – the extracellular deposition of abnormal and insoluble, β-pleated proteinaceous deposits; amyloid causes its pathological effects by accumulating in body tissues.

53   C   Tuberculosis (TB)

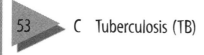

Granulomatous inflammation is a distinctive pattern of chronic inflammation that is characterised by granuloma formation and usually occurs in response to the presence of indigestible matter within macrophages.

Histologically, a granuloma consists of a microscopic aggregation of activated macrophages that are transformed into epithelium-like cells (epithelioid macrophages), surrounded by a collar of mononuclear leukocytes, principally lymphocytes and occasionally plasma cells. Epithelioid cells may coalesce to form multinucleate giant cells. Their nuclei are often arranged around the periphery of the cell – Langerhans' giant cells. Do not confuse the term 'granuloma' with 'granulation tissue' – the latter is a wound-healing phenomenon and does not include granulomas.

TB is the archetypal granulomatous disease, but it can also occur in other disease states, such as other infections (eg leprosy, schistosomiasis), or with foreign bodies, which may be endogenous (bone, adipose tissue, uric acid crystals) or exogenous (eg silica, suture materials). Some causes are idiopathic, such as Crohn's disease and sarcoidosis. Note that Crohn's disease, but not ulcerative colitis, is associated with the presence of granulomas. Lobar pneumonia and bronchopneumonia do not characteristically form granulomas.

If the granuloma is large it may outstrip its own blood supply, resulting in central necrosis. TB is characteristically associated with caseating granulomas, with central caseous necrosis. Other conditions, such as Crohn's disease and sarcoidosis, are associated with non-caseating granulomas.

54   A   Granulation tissue actively contracts

The stages of wound healing are as follows:

- coagulation/haemostasis (immediate)

- inflammation (0–4 days): initially neutrophils and then macrophages, which remove tissue debris

- fibroplasia and epithelialisation (4 days to 3 weeks): neovascularised tissue known as granulation tissue

- contraction, maturation and remodelling (3 weeks to 18 months): fibroblasts differentiate into myofibroblasts, which are responsible for active wound contraction; maximal wound tensile strength is achieved at about day 60, when it is 80% of normal.

Resolution is the most favourable outcome of the healing process because it refers to the complete restitution of normal tissue architecture and function. It can occur only if tissue damage is slight, followed by rapid removal of debris. No scar tissue forms in pure resolution.

Repair, on the other hand, is the replacement of damaged tissue by fibrosis or gliosis, which fills or bridges the defect, but has no intrinsic specialised function relevant to the organ in which repair occurs. It occurs when there is substantial damage to the specialised connective tissue framework and/or the tissue lacks the ability to regenerate specialised cells. The result of repair is a scar.

Tissue repair occurs through the formation of granulation tissue. It derives its name from the granular appearance seen by early military surgeons in the base of wounds that were about to heal, hence the association with a favourable outcome. The granules are caused by the sprouting of endothelial buds as a result of angiogenesis. Granulation tissue replaces a disorganised mess by orderly new fibrous tissue, a process called organisation. Granulation tissue should not be confused with granulomas (aggregates of activated macrophages), which are not an integral part of granulation tissue.

Granulation tissue is defined by the presence of three cell types:

1. Macrophages: responsible for removing tissue debris

2. Fibroblasts: responsible for laying down the collagen in fibrous tissue that aids wound contraction

3. Endothelial cells: responsible for the formation of new blood vessels (angiogenesis).

Lymphocytes and plasma cells may also be present.

Healing by primary intention refers to incised wounds where the edges can be apposed. Healing by secondary intention is where there has been tissue loss and the edges cannot be suitably apposed. Healing by secondary intention is slower because granulation tissue has to form from the base of the wound and re-epithelialisation has to occur from the edges to cover this. The granulation tissue eventually contracts, resulting in scar formation.

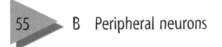

55   B   Peripheral neurons

The cells of the body are divided into three groups on the basis of their proliferative capacity:

1. Continuously dividing cells (self-renewing or labile cells) continue to proliferate throughout life. This includes surface epithelia and cells of the bone marrow. Bone has excellent properties of regeneration and remodelling of a fractured callus can produce complete restoration of a fractured bone.

2. Quiescent (or stable) cells normally demonstrate a low level of replication. However, they can undergo rapid division in response to stimuli and are thus capable of reconstituting the tissue of origin. They are considered to be in G_0 of the cell cycle but can be stimulated into G_1. In this category are the parenchymal cells of virtually all the glandular organs of the body, best exemplified by the ability of the liver to regenerate after hepatectomy or toxic, viral or chemical injury. However, regeneration does not necessarily mean restoration of normal structure. Thus, if damage to the liver continues while replication occurs, there may not be a complete return to the original architecture and if the damage is severe cirrhosis may result.

3. Non-dividing (or permanent) cells have left the cell cycle and cannot replicate so that regeneration is not possible. Neurons of the CNS (brain and spinal cord) and skeletal and cardiac myocytes belong to this group. That these cells cannot regenerate probably reflects the fact that the spatial organisation of these tissues is so specific that regeneration would result in functional chaos. The result is that damaged areas of cardiac muscle are replaced by fibrous scar tissue after a myocardial infarction.

ANSWERS

Principles of pathology – Answers

The absence of regeneration within the CNS reflects not only the intrinsic properties of the neurons themselves, which are incapable of dividing, but also the inhibitory environment present within the CNS. Under normal circumstances, the physiological purpose of the inhibitory environment present within the CNS is to prevent the formation of unwanted connections and help to maintain the structural integrity of white matter tracts. However, this is detrimental in the setting of injury. Thus, gliosis is the only reaction that the brain and spinal cord can make after injury and the inability of central neurons to regenerate may result in permanent loss of function (eg permanent paralysis in the case of spinal cord trauma).

Peripheral nerves, on the other hand, unlike their CNS counterparts, are able to regenerate after injury, with axonal growth occurring at a rate of about 1 mm/day. A better understanding of why regenerative capacity is so much greater in the peripheral nervous system than the CNS may open up new therapeutic windows for repairing the damaged CNS in patients for whom there is currently little hope.

C Is classically liquefactive necrosis in the brain

Necrosis is abnormal tissue death during life. Necrosis is always pathological and accompanied by inflammation. Groups of cells are involved and undergo swelling and lysis. Necrotic cells are phagocytosed by inflammatory cells. There are several different types of necrosis:

- Coagulative (structured) necrosis: the most common form of necrosis. Results from interruption of the blood supply. Tissue architecture is preserved. Seen in organs supplied by end-arteries such as the kidney, heart, liver, spleen.

- Liquefactive (colliquative) necrosis: occurs in tissues rich in lipid where lysosomal enzymes denature the fat and cause liquefaction of the tissue. Characteristically occurs in the brain.

- Caseous (unstructured) necrosis: gross appearance is of soft, cheesy friable material. Tissue architecture is destroyed. Commonly seen in TB.

- Fat necrosis: can occur after direct trauma (eg breast) or enzymatic lipolysis (eg pancreatitis).

- Fibrinoid necrosis: seen in the walls of arteries that are subjected to high pressures as in malignant hypertension. The muscular wall undergoes necrosis and is associated with deposition of fibrin.

- Gangrenous necrosis: this is irreversible tissue death characterised by putrefaction. It may be wet, dry or gaseous. The tissues appear green or black because of the breakdown of haemoglobin.

ANSWERS

Principles of pathology – Answers

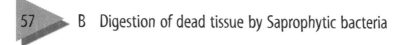

In gangrene, tissue that is dead is digested by bacteria that are incapable of invading and multiplying in living tissue (saprophytes), a process known as putrefaction. Gas production may be present in some forms of gangrene (eg gas gangrene from clostridial anaerobic infection), but not others.

Necrosis of tissue is an essential prerequisite for gangrene. It may, however, be caused by ischaemia (secondary gangrene or dry gangrene) or bacterial toxins (primary gangrene or wet [moist] gangrene).

A thrombus is solid material formed from the constituents of flowing blood. Three primary influences predispose to thrombus formation, the so-called Virchow's triad.

Virchow's triad

1. Damaged vessel wall: denuded endothelium

2. Changes in blood flow – turbulence, stasis

3. Alterations in blood constituents: platelets, clotting factors, blood, hyperlipidaemia, hyperviscosity, etc.

The normal, intact endothelium is anti-thrombotic. This prevents the clotting of blood within the normal circulation. When the endothelium is injured, thrombosis occurs. Under physiological circumstances this prevents haemorrhage, as part of the normal haemostatic response to injury. Only when the formation of thrombus becomes excessive does it become pathological, resulting in vascular obstruction or migration of the thrombus to a distant site (embolisation).

Heparin and warfarin both reduce the risk of thrombosis by their action on the clotting cascade. Thrombocytopenia means a low platelet count, which also reduces the risk of thrombosis. Increased blood viscosity increases the risk of thrombosis ('thicker blood clots more easily'). Immobility increases the risk of thrombosis by stasis.

ANSWERS

Principles of pathology – Answers

E   Generally has a worse outcome than a thrombus

A thrombus is an organised mass of blood constituents that forms in flowing blood (ie in the living body).

A clot is a solid mass of blood constituents formed in stationary blood when blood is allowed to coagulate outside the body or post mortem.

An embolus is an abnormal mass of undissolved material (of solid, liquid or gaseous origin) that is carried in the bloodstream from one place to another.

Thrombus and clot can be readily distinguished from each other post mortem:

Thrombus	Post mortem clot
Grey	Dark purple–red
Organised structure forming lines of Zahn (the pale lines are platelet aggregates enmeshed in fibrin, whereas the intervening dark lines are made up of red blood cells)	Separation of red blood cells and plasma producing a 'chicken-fat' appearance because red cells often gravitate to the bottom of a post mortem clot
Dull surface and firm consistency	Shiny surface and gelatinous consistency ('redcurrant jelly')
Adheres to the vessel wall	Peels away easily from the vessel wall
Dry, granular and friable	Moist and rubbery
Conforms to shape of vessel	Does not conform to shape of vessel
May show features of recanalisation	

Veins, rather than arteries, are the most common source of emboli, which most commonly arise from thrombosis formed within the deep veins of the lower limb and pelvis; thrombus formed here is known as a deep vein thrombosis. Anatomy ensures that emboli of venous origin lodge in pulmonary arteries. The size of the pulmonary artery blocked depends on the size of the thromboembolus. Usually thromboemboli are small and lodge in small pulmonary arteries, although sometimes an extensive thrombus from the deep veins ends up as a saddle embolus blocking the main pulmonary artery. This massive pulmonary embolus is the most common preventable cause of death in hospitalised, bed-bound patients.

An embolus is not always a result of thrombus, although about 95% of all emboli are thrombotic. Other emboli include:

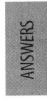

- solid material: fat, tumour cells, atheromatous material, foreign matter
- liquid material: amniotic fluid
- gas material: air, nitrogen bubbles.

The ischaemia resulting from an embolus tends to be worse than that caused by thrombosis because the blockage is so sudden. Thrombi tend to occlude the vessel lumen slowly, so they are less likely to cause infarction because they provide time for the development of alternative perfusion pathways via collaterals.

60 ▸ C Is an abnormal reduction of the blood supply to or drainage from an organ or tissue

- Ischaemia is an abnormal reduction of the blood supply to or drainage from an organ or tissue.

- Infarction is the death of tissues specifically caused by ischaemia or loss of blood supply.

- Necrosis refers to generalised tissue death caused by toxins, trauma or vascular occlusion.

Ischaemia is most commonly the result of vascular narrowing or occlusion from atherosclerosis. However, the blood supply to tissues may be inadequate for a variety of reasons other than vascular occlusion. Thus, ischaemia may also be the result of states of shock (ie circulatory collapse with low arterial blood pressure). The most common causes of shock are insufficient blood volume (hypovolaemia), sepsis and heart failure. In all cases there is a low blood pressure. All tissues may therefore become ischaemic and any organ may fail.

The outcome of ischaemia is determined by a variety of different factors:

- The nature of the vascular supply: the most important factor. The presence of collaterals is protective against the effects of ischaemia. Conversely blockage of an end-artery will almost always cause infarction.

- The tissue involved: the brain and heart are more susceptible to the effects of hypoxia.

- The speed of onset: slowly developing occlusions are less likely to cause infarction because they provide time for the development of alternative perfusion pathways.

- The degree of obstruction and the calibre of the vessel occluded.

- The oxygen content of the blood supplying the ischaemic tissue.

- The presence of concomitant heart failure.

- The state of the microcirculation as in diabetes mellitus.

61   C   Induces acute inflammatory changes, maximal at 1–3 days after the infarct

Myocardial infarction is infarction of the myocardium as a result of severe ischaemia leading to necrosis of the myocardium. It is usually the result of coronary artery occlusion secondary to atherosclerosis, with or without superimposed thrombosis or plaque haemorrhage.

Only rarely is a myocardial infarct the result of an embolic event. In at least 10% of patients myocardial infarction is painless or 'silent'; this is particularly true in people with diabetes and elderly patients because of the accompanying autonomic neuropathy.

If a patient survives an acute infarction, the infarct heals through the formation of scar tissue. The infarcted tissue is not replaced by new cardiac muscle because cardiac myocytes are permanent (non-dividing) cells and cardiac muscle is therefore unable to regenerate. Scar tissue does not possess the usual contractile properties of normal cardiac muscle; the result is contractile dysfunction or congestive cardiac failure.

The macroscopic and microscopic changes of myocardial infarcts follow a predictable sequence of events. The chief features are coagulative necrosis and inflammatory cell infiltration, followed by organisation and repair where granulation tissue replaces dead muscle and is gradually converted into scar tissue. The entire process from coagulative necrosis to the formation of well-formed scar tissue takes 6–8 weeks.

Time	Macroscopic changes	Microscopic changes
0–12 h	None	None
12–24 h	Infarcted area appears pale with blotchy discoloration	Infarcted muscle brightly eosinophilic with intercellular oedema; beginning of neutrophilic infiltrate
24–72 h	Infarcted area appears soft and pale; mottling with a yellow–tan infarct centre	Coagulation necrosis and acute inflammatory response most prominent; loss of nuclei and striations; marked infiltration by neutrophils
3–10 days	Hyperaemic border develops around the yellow dead muscle	Organisation of infarcted area and replacement with granulation tissue; dying neutrophils with macrophages predominating; disintegration and phagocytosis of dead myofibres
Weeks to months	Tough grey–white scar	Progressive collagen deposition; infarct is replaced by a dense acellular scar

62 **B Most commonly occurs at branching points within the circulation**

Atherosclerosis is a focal disease of the tunica intima of large and medium-sized arteries and consists of the gradual accumulation of focal raised patches (plaques) on the arterial lining, in response to arterial wall injury. Its complications are the main cause of death in urbanised societies.

The anatomical sites of atherosclerosis are somewhat predictable. Plaques generally occur at branching points and bends in arteries exposed to high pressure, with pulmonary arteries being relatively spared and veins completely so. The turbulence and eddy currents set up at branching points expose the intimal surface to haemodynamic injury, and encourage the uptake of circulating lipoproteins and macrophages into the vessel wall. Thus, atherosclerotic plaques are common at sites of bifurcation such as:

ANSWERS

- the entrance to the coronary ostia (causing a myocardial infarction)
- close to where the descending abdominal aorta bifurcates into the common iliac arteries (resulting in an abdominal aortic aneurysm)
- in the internal carotid artery close to where the common carotid bifurcates into internal and external branches (resulting in a cerebrovascular accident)
- close to where the renal arteries break off the aorta (resulting in renal artery stenosis)
- in the iliofemoral arteries of the lower limb (causing lower limb ischaemia).

Principles of pathology – Answers

The lesions are essentially foci of chronic inflammation in which the macrophages seem to be doing harm. The basic lesion, consisting of a raised focal plaque within the intima, has a core of lipid (mainly cholesterol) and a covering fibrous cap.

The four most important risk factors for atherosclerosis to remember are those that are potentially controllable, namely high cholesterol, diabetes mellitus, smoking and hypertension. All are associated with intimal injury and accelerate atherosclerosis. Atherosclerosis is a reversible disease process so that risk factor modification ameliorates the size of atherosclerotic plaques. Risk factor modification forms an essential part of the management of patients with known atherosclerotic disease.

Section B
Therapeutics

Therapeutics
Questions

63 Which of the following is true with regard to local anaesthetics?

○ A Cocaine is an amide

○ B Addition of epinephrine increases systemic absorption of the local anaesthetic

○ C One of the first signs of toxicity is perioral paraesthesia

○ D Local anaesthetics work by blocking potassium channels in the nerve endings

○ E They inhibit the propagation of impulses in Aβ-fibres first

64 Aspirin (acetylsalicylic acid)

○ A Is a lipoxygenase inhibitor

○ B Inhibits the coagulation cascade

○ C Inhibits platelet aggregation

○ D Is a reversible cyclo-oxygenase inhibitor

○ E Works by acetylating an aspartate residue at the active site

65 Aspirin damages the gastric mucosa through which of the following mechanisms?

- A Reduced surface mucus secretion
- B Increased mucosal blood flow
- C Increased surface bicarbonate secretion
- D Reduced acid secretion by gastric parietal cells
- E Delayed gastric emptying

66 With regard to anti-emetics, which of the following is true?

- A Cyclizine acts on the histaminergic system
- B Ondansetron primarily acts on the dopaminergic system
- C Prochlorperazine acts on the cholinergic system
- D Metoclopramide is the drug of choice for motion sickness
- E Metoclopramide is the anti-emetic of choice in Parkinson's disease

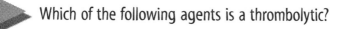 Which of the following agents is a thrombolytic?

- ○ A Warfarin
- ○ B Aspirin
- ○ C Fibrinogen
- ○ D Streptokinase
- ○ E Heparin

 Opioids:

- ○ A Commonly cause diarrhoea
- ○ B Act only centrally
- ○ C Mediate most of their beneficial effects and side effects through σ-receptors
- ○ D Cause tolerance
- ○ E Can be reversed by flumazenil

69 ▶ Which of the following drugs is the most potent inhibitor of gastric acid secretion?

○ A   Chlorphenamine
○ B   Misoprostol
○ C   Ranitidine
○ D   Omeprazole
○ E   Gaviscon

70 ▶ Which one of the following is a depolarising neuromuscular blocker?

○ A   Atracurium
○ B   Atropine
○ C   Guanethidine
○ D   Suxamethonium
○ E   Neostigmine

71 The following are classes of antihypertensive agents except:

○ A ACE inhibitors
○ B β-Blockers
○ C α-Blockers
○ D Angiotensin II receptor antagonists
○ E Calcium channel agonists

72 With regard to antidiabetic agents, which drug stimulates the release of insulin from the pancreas?

○ A Actrapid
○ B Gliclazide
○ C Metformin
○ D Rosiglitazone
○ E Acarbose

73 Which of the following diuretics acts mainly on the distal convoluted tubule to decrease water reabsorption?

○ A Furosemide
○ B Acetazolamide
○ C Bendroflumethiazide
○ D Bumetanide
○ E Vasopressin

74 Which antibiotic acts by inhibiting protein synthesis?

○ A Penicillin
○ B Erythromycin
○ C Cefuroxime
○ D Trimethoprim
○ E Co-trimoxazole

75 Which of the following lipid-lowering agents acts by inhibiting HMG-CoA reductase?

○ A Nicotinic acid
○ B Bezafibrate
○ C Colestyramine
○ D Simvastatin
○ E ω3-fatty acids

76 Which anti-arrhythmic drugs acts by inhibiting potassium channels?

○ A Lidocaine
○ B Atenolol
○ C Amiodarone
○ D Verapamil
○ E Diltiazem

77 Which of the following anti-parkinsonian drugs is a COMT (catechol-O-methyltransferase) inhibitor?

○ A Selegiline
○ B L-Dopa
○ C Entacapone
○ D Benzatropine
○ E Bromocriptine

78 In the treatment of asthma, the drug salbutamol principally acts by which of the following mechanisms?

○ A α_1-Adrenoceptor antagonist
○ B β_1-Adrenoceptor agonist
○ C β_2-Adrenoceptor agonist
○ D β_2-Adrenoceptor antagonist
○ E Muscarinic antagonist

Therapeutics
Answers

63 ▶ **C One of the first signs of toxicity is perioral paraesthesia**

There are two separate classes of local anaesthetics: amides and esters. Amides account for most local anaesthetics in clinical use, although cocaine is an ester. Local anaesthetics work by blocking sodium channels. This prevents depolarisation and thereby propagation of pain impulses along the nerve.

Local anaesthetics tend to block the smaller fibres before the larger ones, ie the smaller pain fibres are blocked first (Aδ-fibres and C-fibres) with sparing of the larger neurons such as the motor fibres.

The addition of epinephrine to local anaesthetic has three effects: first it prevents bleeding by a direct effect of epinephrine on the local vasculature, causing vasoconstriction; second, by way of vasoconstriction, it prevents systemic absorption of the local anaesthetic, thereby preventing toxicity/side effects and increasing the local duration of action; and third, by preventing systemic absorption, it allows larger doses to be used than would otherwise be allowed in the absence of epinephrine. However, because of this 'vasoconstrictive effect' epinephrine must never be used on pedicles that contain an end-artery (eg digits, nose tips, ear lobe, penis, etc) where ischaemic necrosis may result.

It is important that the maximum dose of local anaesthetic not be exceeded otherwise the consequences may be lethal. This is because local anaesthetics are cardiotoxic by blocking sodium channels and interfering with cardiac conduction. One of the earliest and most reliable signs of systemic toxicity is perioral tingling. This may be followed by cardiovascular collapse and death.

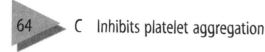

64   C   Inhibits platelet aggregation

Aspirin irreversibly blocks the action of the cyclo-oxygenase enzyme involved in arachidonic acid metabolism, leading to prostaglandin and thromboxane A_2 (TxA_2) production. It does this by acetylating a serine residue at the active site, thereby excluding arachidonic acid. Aspirin has anti-inflammatory, analgesic, antipyretic and antiplatelet actions. All four actions result from the decreased production of prostaglandins and TxA_2.

Aspirin has no effect on the coagulation cascade. The antiplatelet effect of aspirin deserves special mention and is widely used therapeutically in the primary and secondary prevention of cardiovascular and cerebrovascular disease. Aspirin has also recently been shown to have a protective effect against colorectal carcinoma.

The antiplatelet effect of aspirin largely arises through the opposing effects of TxA_2 (produced by platelets) in promoting platelet aggregation and prostaglandin I_2 (PGI_2 or prostacyclin, produced by endothelial cells) in inhibiting platelet aggregation. Aspirin, by inhibiting the cyclo-oxygenase enzyme, results in decreased production of TxA_2 from platelets (thus inhibiting platelet aggregation) and PGI_2 from endothelial cells (thus promoting platelet aggregation).

The TxA_2 effect outweighs the PGI_2 effect, however, for two reasons: first, because aspirin is taken orally, high concentrations of aspirin are found within the portal vein, which results in platelets being exposed to a high concentration of aspirin. This is contrary to endothelial cells, which are in contact with lower concentrations of aspirin once it has been diluted throughout the body and because of pre-systemic metabolism of aspirin to salicylate by esterases in the liver. Second, platelets have no nuclei. This means that, once cyclo-oxygenase is inhibited, production is abolished for the rest of the platelet's lifespan. TxA_2 synthesis does not therefore recover until the affected cohort of platelets is replaced in 7–10 days. Endothelial cells, on the other hand, are nucleated and so able to re-synthesise new cyclo-oxygenase enzyme (and therefore PGI_2).

65 A Reduced surface mucus secretion

Within the normal gastric epithelium, there is a fine balance between normal damaging forces (such as gastric acidity and peptic enzymes) and various protective mechanisms (such as surface mucus production, bicarbonate secretion, mucosal blood flow, elaboration of prostaglandins, tight junctions between cells, epithelial regenerative capacity).

Any disruption of this fine balance, either as a result of increased damaging forces or through impaired defences, may cause epithelial damage and formation of a peptic ulcer. One of the main drawbacks of aspirin is the risk of gastric erosions and peptic ulcer disease associated with its use. This is principally brought about through the following mechanisms:

- a direct irritant effect of aspirin
- a reduction in PGE_2 (which normally serves to increase

local mucus and bicarbonate secretion, thereby protecting the gastric mucosal lining)

- a reduction in PGI_2 (thereby resulting in reduced blood flow to the gastric lining and mucosal ischaemia, preventing the elimination of acid that has diffused into the submucosa)

- increased acid production from gastric parietal cells (prostaglandins normally inhibit acid secretion)

- the antiplatelet effect of aspirin, which propagates any bleeding that may result from an already injured gastric mucosal surface.

Aspirin has no effect on gastric motility. Patients aged over 65, or those with a history of a previous peptic ulcer, should have a proton pump inhibitor (such as omeprazole) co-administered with aspirin. This has been shown to reduce the risk of gastrointestinal bleeding and peptic ulceration.

66   A   Cyclizine acts on the histaminergic system

Antiemetics are drugs that are used clinically to suppress the vomiting reflex. This is mediated primarily through their suppressive effect at specialised sites within the central nervous system (CNS) wherein the vomiting reflex is mediated, namely the vomiting centre, chemoreceptor trigger zone in the area postrema (an area of the brain that is devoid of blood–brain barrier and so in direct contact with emetogenic chemicals within the bloodstream) and the vestibular system (explains motion sickness).

A vast array of drugs is used within the clinical setting, all of which act at different sites within the nervous system and on different neurochemical systems, and yet all result in a similar desired effect (ie suppression of vomiting). The clinical importance of this is pharmacological synergy, namely the additive effect of two different antiemetics used in combination is greater than the sum of the two separate effects because of the different mechanisms of action. It also allows the astute clinician to pick and choose an antiemetic (and thereby a mode of action) that conforms well to a specified clinical scenario.

Chemical neurotransmitter	Examples of drugs
Acetylcholine	Anticholinergics (eg hyoscine)
Histamine	Antihistamines (eg cyclizine)
5-Hydroxytryptamine (5-HT or serotonin)	5-HT_3-receptor antagonists (eg ondansetron, granisetron)
Dopamine	Dopamine antagonists (eg metoclopramide, domperidone, prochlorperazine)

A good example is motion sickness, which seems to depend upon the influential effect of the environment on the vestibular system; the effects of this are, in turn, mediated through the cholinergic system. It is thus easy to see why hyoscine is the most efficacious drug in the setting of motion sickness, but is less efficacious in other situations. Dopamine antagonists, such as metoclopramide, and 5-HT_3 antagonists are ineffective in the treatment or prevention of motion sickness. Similarly, domperidone is the drug of choice in Parkinson's disease because domperidone is a dopamine antagonist that does not cross the blood–brain barrier; if, however, metoclopramide were to be used instead (also a dopamine antagonist, but does cross the blood–brain barrier) symptoms of Parkinson's disease would be exacerbated.

ANSWERS

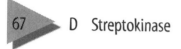

67 ▶ D Streptokinase

Thrombolytics are substances that break down fibrin (fibrinolytics).

Streptokinase is used as a therapeutic fibrinolytic agent in the management of acute myocardial infarction. Warfarin prevents the formation of thrombus by decreasing the amount of vitamin K-dependent clotting factors, although it does not possess fibrinolytic activity. Heparin potentiates the action of antithrombin and also prevents the formation of thrombus, but has no fibrinolytic activity. Aspirin is an antiplatelet agent that acts by reducing the aggregation of platelets. Fibrinogen is a precursor of fibrin, which is involved in the formation of thrombus.

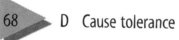

68 ▶ D Cause tolerance

Opioids are mainly used in the hospital setting for their analgesic properties. They are now believed to act both peripherally (outside the CNS) and within the CNS itself.

Unfortunately opioids exert most of their beneficial effects and side effects through the same opioid receptor (μ-receptor). It is therefore unlikely that we will ever be able to develop a synthetic opioid agent that has the analgesic properties of other opioids without their unpleasant side effects.

Constipation and nausea and vomiting are common side effects of opioids. It is therefore always a good idea to co-prescribe laxatives and antiemetics whenever an opioid is prescribed. Opioids cause tolerance, dependence and withdrawal with increasing use. Tolerance means that increasing dosages of the drug need to be used in order to obtain the same effect.

It is important to know how to reverse the effects of opioids because opioid overdose may be fatal. Specific opioid antagonists include naloxone and naltrexone. Flumazenil antagonises the effects of benzodiazepines.

Opioids induce side effects through both excitatory and inhibitory mechanisms

Excitatory effects:

- Pinpoint pupils (direct effect of opioids on the Edinger–Westphal nucleus)
- Nausea and vomiting (direct effect on the area postrema)
- Pruritus (caused by mast cell degranulation and histamine release)
- Dysphoria and euphoria (direct effect on the CNS).

Inhibitory effects:

- Cardiorespiratory depression
- Sedation
- Relaxation of smooth muscles – constipation, urinary retention.

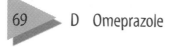

69 ▶ D Omeprazole

Three main classes of drugs are used to combat gastric hyperacidity. From least to most potent they are:

1. Antacids

2. H_2-receptor antagonists

3. Proton pump inhibitors (PPIs).

Only the H_2-receptor antagonists and PPIs reduce the secretion of acid from parietal cells. Of these the PPIs (eg omeprazole and lansoprazole) are the most potent and have the longest duration of action. The reasons for this are twofold: first, PPIs target the terminal stage in gastric acid secretion, namely the proton pump, which is directly responsible for secreting H^+ ions into the gastric lumen; and, second, the irreversible nature of proton pump inhibition means that acid secretion resumes only after the synthesis of new enzyme. PPIs are extremely effective in promoting ulcer healing, even in patients who are resistant to H_2-receptor antagonists.

H_2-receptor antagonists should not, however, be regarded as obsolete because they have a faster onset of action compared with PPIs, but they are less potent in inhibiting gastric acid secretion and have a relatively short duration of action. H_2-receptor antagonists (eg cimetidine and ranitidine) competitively inhibit histamine actions at all H_2-receptors. Acid secretion is not mediated via H_1-receptors and therefore chlorphenamine has no effect on acid secretion.

Antacids have no effect on the secretion of gastric acid from parietal cells, but exert their effect by neutralising the acid that is produced. Their efficacy is limited because the rise in pH stimulates gastrin secretion, which in turn stimulates more acid release (the 'acid rebound effect'). This effect does not occur

ANSWERS

MCQs in Applied Basic Sciences for Medical Students: Volume 2

with H_2-receptor antagonists and PPIs, which act directly on parietal cells. Alginates (eg Gaviscon) are sometimes used and are believed to increase adherence of mucus to the mucosa, thereby increasing mucosal resistance to acid pepsin attack.

Misoprostol is a synthetic prostaglandin analogue that promotes ulcer healing by stimulating protective mechanisms in the gastric mucosa (increased mucus, bicarbonate and blood flow) and by reducing acid secretion. It is sometimes co-administered with non-steroidal anti-inflammatory drugs (NSAIDs) in elderly people to prevent peptic ulcer disease. However, misoprostol is not as efficacious as a PPI and use is limited by its tendency to cause troublesome diarrhoea.

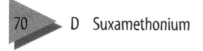

Neuromuscular blockers are commonly used drugs in anaesthesia. By specific blockade of the neuromuscular junction (NMJ) they relax skeletal muscles and induce paralysis. This enables light levels of anaesthesia to be employed with adequate relaxation of the muscles of the abdomen and diaphragm, thereby facilitating surgery.

Neuromuscular blockers also relax the vocal folds and allow the easy passage of a tracheal tube at anaesthetic induction – a procedure known as endotracheal intubation. They can be used only when mechanical ventilation is available because such drugs also paralyse the main muscles of respiration. Neuromuscular blockers can be divided into two main types: depolarising and non-depolarising blockers.

Non-depolarising blockers (eg atracurium), also known as competitive muscle relaxants, compete with acetylcholine for receptor sites at the NMJ and their action can be reversed with anticholinesterases, such as neostigmine. Atropine is a muscarinic antagonist and is often given with neostigmine in order to prevent the muscarinic (parasympathomimetic) side effects of anticholinesterases (such as bradycardia, excessive salivation).

Depolarising blockers (eg suxamethonium, also known as succinylcholine) act by mimicking the action of acetylcholine at the NMJ, but hydrolysis is much slower than for acetylcholine because it is resistant to degradation by cholinesterase. Depolarisation is therefore prolonged, resulting in sodium channel inactivation and neuromuscular blockade. Unlike non-depolarising agents, its action cannot be reversed and recovery is spontaneous. Indeed, anticholinesterases such as neostigmine potentiate the neuromuscular block. Anticholinesterases are also used in myasthenia gravis to enhance neuromuscular transmission by prolonging the action of acetylcholine.

Suxamethonium has a half-life of only a few minutes and is rapidly hydrolysed by the enzyme pseudocholinesterase. In patients with deficient or atypical pseudocholinesterase (an autosomal recessive condition), metabolism is reduced and the half-life and duration of action of suxamethonium are prolonged, resulting in 'scoline apnoea', or prolonged paralysis. Assisted ventilation should be continued until muscle function has been restored. In addition, suxamethonium may also be responsible for triggering malignant hyperthermia in susceptible individuals – an autosomal dominant disorder that results in intense muscular spasm and hyperpyrexia, and is associated with a high mortality.

Guanethidine inhibits the release of norepinephrine from postganglionic sympathetic nerve terminals. It has largely fallen out of use but is extremely effective in lowering blood pressure and may be useful in cases of resistant hypertension.

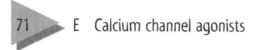

71 ▶ E   Calcium channel agonists

The following classes of antihypertensive drugs are currently in use (remembered by AAABCD):

- ACE (angiotensin-converting enzyme) inhibitors
- angiotensin II receptor antagonists
- α blockers
- β blockers
- calcium channel blockers (antagonists)
- diuretics.

Lowering raised blood pressure has successfully been shown (in both primary and secondary preventive settings) to reduce the risk of stroke, coronary events, heart failure and renal failure. The choice of antihypertensive drug will depend on the relevant indications or contraindications for the individual patient. In addition, a single agent may not be enough and additional blood pressure-lowering drugs may have to be added until the blood pressure is well controlled.

α-Blockers have largely been superseded by other classes of antihypertensive agents. However, they still play an important role in the management of phaeochromocytoma (an epinephrine-secreting tumour of the adrenal medulla). In such instances α-receptors must be blocked before β-receptor blockade to prevent a dangerous hypertensive crisis developing.

Angiotensin II receptor antagonists are generally used as second-line agents when patients are unable to tolerate an ACE inhibitor. Of patients taking ACE inhibitors 15–30% develop an intractable cough, which is believed to result from the accumulation of bradykinin (angiotensin-converting enzyme normally assists in the degradation of bradykinin and its derivatives). In such cases the patient may benefit from conversion to an angiotensin II receptor antagonist.

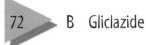

72 ► B   Gliclazide

Sulphonylureas (gliclazide and glibenclamide) are indicated when diet fails to control hyperglycaemia. They stimulate insulin release from the pancreas and are therefore of use only in patients who still have residual pancreatic islet cell function. Side effects include weight gain and hypoglycaemia.

Metformin increases the sensitivity to insulin at the receptor level, but should be avoided in patients with impaired renal function. Side effects include lactic acidosis, nausea, vomiting and diarrhoea.

Rosiglitazone is an example of a thiazolidinedione. This class of drugs acts by increasing the sensitivity of insulin through binding to a nuclear receptor called PPAR-γ. It is not a first-line treatment and should be used in combination with metformin or a sulphonylurea. Rosiglitazone is currently contraindicated in heart failure because it is thought to worsen this condition.

Acarbose acts by delaying the digestion and absorption of starch and sucrose, through the inhibition of intestinal α-glucosidases. Its main side effect is flatulence.

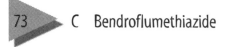

Thiazide diuretics, which include bendroflumethiazide and metolazone, act mainly on the distal convoluted tubule where sodium reabsorption is inhibited. Water accompanies the sodium.

Common side effects include hypokalaemia, hyperuricaemia and impaired glucose tolerance. Potassium loss arises from two distinct mechanisms that are not mutually exclusive. First, an increased sodium load in the collecting ducts stimulates sodium absorption in exchange for potassium secretion. Second, the high flow rate of filtrate produced by these diuretics will also favour potassium excretion by continually flushing it away, increasing the gradient from cell to lumen.

Acetazolamide is a carbonic anhydrase inhibitor, which acts by reducing bicarbonate reabsorption from the proximal tubule. Excretion of bicarbonate, sodium and water is therefore increased.

Furosemide is a loop diuretic that inhibits sodium and chloride reabsorption from the thick ascending loop of Henle (acting on the $Na^+/K^+/2Cl^-$ transporter). Similar to thiazide diuretics, its side effects include hypokalaemia, hyperglycaemia and hyperuricaemia. Bumetanide is also a loop diuretic that behaves in a similar fashion to Frusemide.

Vasopressin (antidiuretic hormone or ADH) acts by increasing the number of aquaporins, or water channels, in the collecting ducts, which in turn increases the reabsorption of water.

Potassium-sparing diuretics (such as spironolactone and amiloride) also act on the distal convoluted tubule and collecting ducts to reduce sodium reabsorption and subsequently water reabsorption. Aldosterone stimulates sodium and subsequent water reabsorption from the distal convoluted tubule.

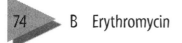
Penicillins and cephalosporins (which include cefuroxime, cefotaxime and ceftriaxone) inhibit bacterial cell wall synthesis through the inhibition of peptidoglycan cross-linking. This weakens bacterial cell walls and renders them susceptible to osmotic shock.

Macrolides (such as erythromycin), tetracyclines, aminoglycosides and chloramphenicol act by interfering with bacterial protein synthesis. Sulphonamides, (such as trimethoprim and co-trimoxazole) work by inhibiting the synthesis of nucleic acid.

Mechanism of action	Examples
Inhibition of cell wall synthesis	Penicillins, cephalosporins, vancomycin
Inhibition of protein synthesis	Macrolides, tetracyclines, aminoglycosides, chloramphenicol, clindamycin
Inhibition of nucleic acid synthesis	Sulphonamides, trimethoprim, quinolones, metronidazole, rifampicin
Inhibition of cell membrane synthesis	Lincomycins, polymyxins

ANSWERS

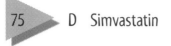

75 ▷ D Simvastatin

Statins reduce cholesterol by competitively inhibiting HMG-CoA (hyroxymethylglutaryl coenzyme A) reductase, an enzyme involved in cholesterol biosynthesis. They are more effective at lowering both total and low-density lipoprotein (LDL) cholesterol than other classes of drugs, but are less effective than fibrates in reducing triglycerides. Side effects include myopathy and deranged liver function.

Nicotinic acid acts by inhibiting the release of very-low-density lipoprotein (VLDL), lowering plasma triglycerides and cholesterol, and increasing high-density lipoprotein (HDL). Its side effects include dizziness and flushing, which limits its use.

Fibrates stimulate lipoprotein lipase activity and work mainly to decrease triglycerides as well as moderately decreasing LDL cholesterol and increasing HDL cholesterol.

Colestyramine (and other anion exchange resins) act by increasing the excretion of bile acids, so more cholesterol is converted into bile acid.

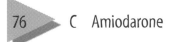

This question requires knowledge of Vaughan Williams' classification of anti-arrhythmic drugs. Lidocaine is a class 1B drug and blocks sodium channels. Procainamide, a class 1A drug, and flecainide, a class 1C drug, also block sodium channels. All class I drugs have membrane-stabilising properties.

Class II drugs comprise the β-blockers. They are believed to work by blocking the pro-arrhythmic effects of catecholamines and the sympathetic nervous system.

Class III drugs (such as amiodarone and sotalol) act through the blockade of potassium channels. They work by prolonging the action potential, thereby increasing the refractory period and, hence, suppressing ectopic and re-entrant activity. Note that sotalol has both class II and class III actions.

Class IV drugs include those such as verapamil and diltiazem that act by blocking calcium channels.

ANSWERS

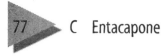

77   C   Entacapone

Parkinson's disease is a progressive neurodegenerative disorder characterised clinically by a triad of bradykinesia, rigidity and resting tremor. It results from the decreased production of dopamine from the substantia nigra of the basal ganglia. Direct replacement with dopamine is not possible because dopamine does not cross the blood–brain barrier.

L-Dopa (levodopa) is the amino acid precursor of dopamine, and is able to cross the blood–brain barrier, where it is converted (decarboxylated) to dopamine. It acts by directly replenishing depleted striatal dopamine. It is given with a dopa decarboxylase inhibitor (eg carbidopa), which does not cross the blood–brain barrier. This reduces the peripheral conversion of L-dopa to dopamine, thereby limiting side effects such as nausea, vomiting and cardiovascular effects (particularly hypotension).

Bromocriptine, cabergoline, ropinirole and pergolide are all dopamine agonists. They may be used alone or in combination with L-dopa.

Selegiline inhibits the enzyme, MAO-B (monoamine oxidase B) for which dopamine is a substrate. It reduces the metabolism of dopamine in the brain and potentiates the action of L-dopa.

Entacapone inhibits the enzyme, COMT, and by so doing it slows the elimination of L-dopa. It prolongs the duration of a single dose, in addition to smoothing out any fluctuations in the plasma concentration of L-dopa.

Muscarinic antagonists, such as benzatropine, may play a role in the management of Parkinson's disease and are particularly useful when resting tremor is the predominant symptom.

ANSWERS

MCQs in Applied Basic Sciences for Medical Students: Volume 2

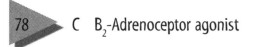

78

C B_2-Adrenoceptor agonist

Asthma is an inflammatory (reactive) disorder of the airways characterised by reversible airway obstruction (or bronchospasm). It results from a type I hypersensitivity reaction, where the IgE-mediated degranulation of mast cells and release of inflammatory mediators are central to the pathogenesis.

Bronchial smooth muscle contains β_2-adrenoceptors. Throughout the body β_2-adrenoceptors act to relax smooth muscle. Salbutamol stimulates these receptors (ie they are selective β_2-adrenoceptor agonists), thereby relaxing the smooth muscle in the airways and increasing their calibre. Longer-acting β_2-adrenoceptor agonists (such as salmeterol) play a role in more severe asthma.

Bronchial smooth muscle also contains muscarinic receptors. Stimulation of these receptors causes smooth muscle contraction, so muscarinic antagonists (such as ipratropium) are useful adjuncts in the management of asthma.

Other drugs used in the management of asthma include steroids (oral or inhaled), leukotriene receptor antagonists (such as montelukast), xanthines (such as theophylline) and sodium cromoglicate.

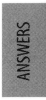

ANSWERS

Therapeutics – Answers

Section C
Cellular biology and clinical genetics

Cellular biology and clinical genetics
Questions

79

With regard to organelles:

○ A   Smooth endoplasmic reticulum makes polypeptides

○ B   Mitochondria perform anaerobic respiration

○ C   Mitochondria can multiply independently

○ D   Prokaryotic cells have membrane-bound organelles

○ E   The Golgi apparatus is involved in the degradation of proteins

80 ► Which of the following is a technique used to identify specific sequences of DNA?

○ A Northern blotting

○ B Southern blotting

○ C Polymerase chain reaction (PCR)

○ D Western blotting

○ E Reverse transcription PCR

81 ► With regard to gene expression, which statement is true:

○ A Translation occurs in the nucleus of eukaryotes

○ B Introns code for proteins

○ C DNA polymerases manufacture DNA in a 3' to 5' direction

○ D RNA polymerase II gives rise to protein-encoding mRNA

○ E Codons are formed from groups of three amino acids

82 With regard to cell division, which of the following is correct?

○ A Transfer of genetic information between homologous chromosomes occurs in metaphase I of meiosis

○ B Mitosis always produces genetically identical daughter cells

○ C Mitosis is controlled externally by cyclins

○ D Cyclins are activated by dephosphorylation

○ E *p53* is an oncogene

 83 With regard to DNA:

○ A Adenine pairs only with thymine

○ B Cytosine always pairs with guanine

○ C The DNA double helix has 12 base-pairs per turn

○ D Uracil is an example of a purine base

○ E All bases are paired by two non-covalent hydrogen bonds

Gene transcription is initiated by:

- ○ A Exons
- ○ B Promoters
- ○ C Silencers
- ○ D Introns
- ○ E Enhancers

A disease inherited as an autosomal dominant disorder:

- ○ A Requires that both parents carry the abnormality
- ○ B Usually prevents reproduction
- ○ C Affects males and females equally
- ○ D Affects all the children of the affected adult
- ○ E May be transmitted by a carrier who does not manifest the disease

86 Which of the following is an autosomal dominant disorder?

○ A Christmas disease
○ B Phenylketonuria
○ C Haemophilia A
○ D Cystic fibrosis
○ E Marfan syndrome

87 A teenager would like genetic counselling. His mother has phenylketonuria or PKU (which is inherited as autosomal recessive). He has a brother with PKU. What is the chance that he is a carrier of the disease?

○ A 0%
○ B 25%
○ C 50%
○ D 75%
○ E 100%

88 Which of the following karyotypes is associated with short stature?

○ A 45XO

○ B 46YO

○ C 46XO

○ D 47XYY

○ E 47XXY

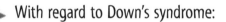

89 With regard to Down's syndrome:

○ A Alzheimer's disease is seen in all individuals with the condition by the age of 45

○ B It is caused by trisomy 23

○ C It most commonly results from a chromosomal translocation

○ D The risk of having a child with Down's syndrome is about 1 in 1000 if the mother is aged 30 years

○ E Individuals with this condition most commonly die prematurely from lung cancer

90 ► Huntington's disease:

○ A Is an autosomal recessive condition
○ B Is a CTG trinucleotide repeat disorder
○ C Causes polyglutamine repeats within the fibrillin protein
○ D Is characterised clinically by a triad of bradykinesia, rigidity and tremor
○ E Exhibits a genetic phenomenon known as 'anticipation'

91 ► With regard to cystic fibrosis:

○ A Inheritance of cystic fibrosis is sex linked
○ B It is caused by a genetic defect on chromosome 6
○ C It is the most common inherited disease in white people
○ D Patients can expect a normal life expectancy
○ E Gene therapy is a well-established treatment option

Cellular biology and clinical genetics – Questions

Haemophilia A:

○ A Is more common in females than in males
○ B Is caused by an abnormal gene on the Y chromosome
○ C Is synonymous with Christmas disease
○ D Is the result of a deficiency in factor IX
○ E Affects the intrinsic, rather than the extrinsic, pathway
       for blood coagulation

With regard to sickle cell anaemia:

○ A The inheritance pattern is autosomal dominant
○ B Ii is caused by a mutation within the haemoglobin α
       chain
○ C The mutation involved is a valine–alanine substitution
○ D It is more common in regions of the world where
       malaria is endemic
○ E It causes splenomegaly in adulthood

94 Which of the following is true for disorders of haemoglobin?

○ A Sickle cell disease is caused by the decreased production of normal globin

○ B Haemoglobin binds more avidly to oxygen than to carbon monoxide

○ C Defective haem synthesis results in porphyria

○ D Thalassaemia is the result of the production of abnormal globin

○ E Cyanide kills by blocking the interaction between oxygen and haemoglobin

95 ABO blood grouping

○ A Blood group O is the universal recipient

○ B The mode of inheritance is autosomal recessive

○ C Blood group AB is the universal donor

○ D Blood group O is recessive to A and B

○ E Individuals of blood group O are resistant to *Plasmodium vivax*

96 ▶ Adult polycystic kidney disease:

○ A Is inherited as an autosomal recessive condition

○ B Affects only one kidney

○ C Is associated with berry aneurysms of the circle of Willis

○ D Commonly presents at birth

○ E Is caused by a mutation in polycystin-1 in all cases

Cellular biology and clinical genetics

Answers

79   C   Mitochondria can multiply independently

Smooth endoplasmic reticulum (ER) is involved in steroid hormone synthesis, whereas rough ER makes polypeptides. Mitochondria are the key organelles in aerobic respiration. They are able to multiply independently and are thought to have evolved millions of years ago from primitive bacteria (endosymbiotic theory), and therefore contain everything that is required to be self-sufficient, including DNA and ribosomes.

Prokaryotic cells have no membrane-bound organelles; eukaryotic cells have the internal compartmentalisation of organelles, and hence their division of labour (specialisation). The Golgi apparatus has a role in the transportation and modification of proteins, eg the glycosylation to proteins. The lysosomes and proteasomes are involved in the degradation of proteins.

80 ▶ B Southern blotting

The PCR is an amplification process used to amplify small amounts of DNA in order to perform analysis. It does not identify specific sequences. The DNA can then be analysed using Southern blotting. PCR involves synthesising two oligonucleotide primers, ie short segments of RNA, which will bind to the DNA; when added to denatured DNA, they will bind to the DNA and amplify it.

The cycle is continually repeated 20–30 times, resulting in an exponential increase in the quantity of DNA. Reverse transcription PCR (rtPCR) uses RNA; as RNA is too unstable to be used for PCR, it must be converted to a complementary copy of DNA using the enzyme reverse transcriptase, and PCR is then performed.

Southern blotting (named after a man called Southern, and the only blotting method to be eponymous) involves digestion of DNA and denaturation in alkali, creating single strands. A permanent copy of the single strands is made by placing the DNA on a nitrocellulose filter, ie the Southern blot. A target, radioactively labelled DNA fragment is added and will bind to its homologous DNA fragment (if present). The DNA is then washed to remove any unbound DNA, and the hybridised DNA can then be visualised as a band using autoradiography.

Northern blotting is similar to Southern blotting but uses mRNA as the target nucleic acid, rather than DNA. The mRNA can be hybridised to a radiolabelled DNA probe.

Western blotting is used to analyse proteins that are separated by electrophoresis, transferred to nitrocellulose, and reacted with antibody for detection. The names northern and western blotting were used to show that they were analogous to Southern blotting.

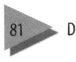

81　D　RNA polymerase II gives rise to protein-encoding mRNA

In prokaryotes transcription and translation occur in the cytoplasm, whereas, in eukaryotes, transcription occurs in the nucleus and translation in the cytoplasm. Transcription is the process of synthesising mRNA from DNA; it is catalysed by the enzyme RNA polymerase II. RNA and DNA is always synthesised in a 5′ to 3′ direction.

The production of mature mRNA is a result of gene splicing. The introns, which are non-coding sequences of DNA, are removed and intervening exons are joined together. The exons are then coded into proteins during translation.

Amino acids are coded for by groups of three bases and each three bases together make up a codon. As there are four types of bases, there is a potential for 4^3 (or 64) amino acids. Only 20 amino acids are used in protein synthesis so in fact 44 codons are considered to be redundant.

82 ▶ **B** Mitosis always produces genetically identical daughter cells

Mitosis is the process of cell division in somatic cells and produces two genetically identical diploid cells. Meiosis occurs in gamete formation and differs from mitosis in two important respects: each daughter cell contains half the genetic information (haploid) and the resultant cells differ in their genetic material.

There are two separate phases (or divisions) in meiosis. In the first division two genetically different haploid cells are formed and in the second each of the haploid cells divides. The exchange of genetic material occurs in prophase I.

The cell cycle is controlled internally by gene products called cyclins, which vary in concentration throughout the cell cycle. Cyclin-dependent kinases control the activity of cyclins by switching them on through phosphorylation. *p53* is an example of a tumour-suppressor gene. It normally functions to inhibit the cell cycle. It is the most commonly mutated gene in cancers. It encodes a transcription factor that downregulates the cell cycle, preventing the cell from undergoing mitosis. Oncogenes control cell growth and differentiation, examples of which include growth factors, growth factor receptors and nuclear transcription factors.

83 ▶ B Cytosine always pairs with guanine

DNA consists of a right-handed double helix with 10 bases per turn. Adenine and guanine are purine bases; cytosine, thymine (and uracil) are pyrimidine bases (remembered by the 'y' in pyrimidine, thymine, cytosine). Adenine pairs with thymine in DNA via two hydrogen bonds and with uracil in RNA. Guanine pairs with cytosine in DNA via three hydrogen bonds.

84 ▶ B Promoters

Transcription of genes is initiated by promoters. Enhancers and silencers are proteins that bind to the promoter region on the DNA and will influence gene transcription. Exons carry the coding sequences of DNA.

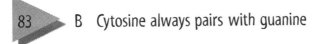

ANSWERS

Cellular biology and clinical genetics – Answers

85 ▸ C Affects males and females equally

Autosomal dominant disorders affect males and females equally because there is no involvement of the sex chromosomes and autosomes are similar for males and females. Only one of the parents needs to carry the abnormality for it to be classified as an autosomal dominant disorder; if both parents were required to carry the abnormality it would be an autosomal recessive disorder.

Only half the children of an affected adult would inherit the condition because half would receive the normal autosome. Carriers of an autosomal dominant trait do not exist, because such carriers exhibit the disease.

Autosomal dominant conditions are commonly transmitted from one generation to the next, either because of their late onset (eg Huntington's disease) or because reproduction occurs before death ensues.

86 ▸ E Marfan syndrome

As a general rule, disorders that affect metabolic pathways/ enzymes are autosomal recessive, whereas diseases that affect structural proteins are autosomal dominant.

Thus, Marfan syndrome, Huntington's disease and neurofibromatosis (von Recklinghausen's disease) are examples of autosomal dominant conditions because they affect structural proteins. Cystic fibrosis and phenylketonuria are autosomal recessive because they affect metabolic pathways.

Haemophilia A, haemophilia B (or Christmas disease) and red–green colour blindness are examples of sex-linked conditions.

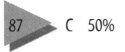

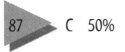

87 **C 50%**

The key to this question is to understand that, in order to have a child with an autosomal recessive disease, both parents must carry the gene, so, although the mother may have the disease, the father has to be a carrier.

The question fails to inform you that the father has the disease, so you can safely assume that he carries only one abnormal gene. To be a carrier for an autosomal recessive disease, you will have one normal and one abnormal copy of the gene. As his mother carries both abnormal genes, and his father carries one abnormal gene and one normal gene, there is a 50% chance that the teenager has the disease and a 50% chance that he is a carrier.

Phenylketonuria, or PKU, is an inborn error of metabolism. As a result of a specific enzyme deficiency, phenylalanine accumulates. The enzyme block leads to a deficiency of tyrosine, in turn leading to a reduction in melanin, so children often have blue eyes and blonde hair. Pigmented areas of the brain are affected, such as the substantia nigra. PKU is tested for at birth in children using the Guthrie test. It can be treated by removing phenylalanine from the diet. If PKU is detected early enough in childhood, learning disabilities can be prevented.

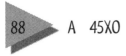

88 **A 45XO**

This is Turner's syndrome – a chromosome disorder caused by the lack of the Y chromosome (45XO). Features include widely spaced nipples, short stature, webbed neck, a kinked aorta (coarctation of aorta), primary amenorrhoea and high arched palate. 47XXY is Klinefelter's syndrome, which is associated with tall stature.

89 ▶ D The risk of having a child with Down's syndrome is about 1 in 1000 if the mother is aged 30 years

Down's syndrome is trisomy 21. It arises in about 1 in 700 births, but there is a strong association between the incidence and advancing maternal age.

When the mother is 30 years old, her risk of having a child with Down's syndrome is 1 in 1000. Affected children have a lower IQ. Classic features include epicanthic folds, a protruding tongue, a single palmar crease, a wide gap between the first and second toe, and cardiac anomalies including atrial and ventricular septal defects. Early death occurs in 15–20% of cases and is usually cardiac related.

A large proportion of, but not all, individuals will develop Alzheimer's disease in later life. This is believed to occur through a gene dosage effect and the accumulation of amyloid precursor protein (the protein linked to Alzheimer's disease), which is coded for by chromosome 21.

The extra chromosome arises in 94% of cases from non-dysjunction at maternal meiosis I. Robertsonian translocations account for 5% of cases and 1% of cases occur as a result of mosaicism.

E Exhibits a genetic phenomenon known as 'anticipation'

Huntington's disease is a late-onset, autosomal dominant disorder characterised by CAG trinucleotide repeat sequences within the huntingtin gene on chromosome 4 (myotonic dystrophy is a CTG trinucleotide repeat disorder). This translates into polyglutamine repeats within the huntingtin protein (not the fibrillin protein, which forms the basis of Marfan syndrome).

Huntington's disease is characterised clinically by a triad of choreiform (dance-like) movements, cognitive changes and psychiatric disturbances. It is Parkinson's disease that is characterised clinically by a triad of bradykinesia, rigidity (which may be of the lead-pipe or cog-wheel variety) and resting tremor. Histologically, Huntington's disease is characterised by atrophy and loss of neurons in the caudate nucleus and putamen.

It is also important to appreciate that Huntington's disease exhibits a genetic phenomenon known as 'anticipation'. This simply means that both the age of onset and severity of the disease phenotype alter with successive generations as a result of the unstable trinucleotide repeat sequence.

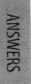

91   C   It is the most inherited disease in white people

Cystic fibrosis (also known as mucoviscidosis) is an autosomal recessive condition, caused by a genetic mutation in the cystic fibrosis transmembrane regulator (CFTR) on chromosome 7. It is the most common inherited disease among white people, affecting 1 in 2500 children. Cystic fibrosis carriers are believed to offer a selective advantage to the population by being relatively more resistant to cholera. This may explain the fact that, on the basis of the frequency of affected homozygotes in the white population, 2–4% must be heterozygote carriers (using the Hardy–Weinberg equation).

Clinical manifestations relate mainly to the lungs (chronic lung infections, especially caused by *Pseudomonas aeruginosa*, bronchiectasis) and the digestive system (meconium ileus, pancreatic insufficiency, failure to thrive). There is no cure for cystic fibrosis. Treatment is mainly supportive, through a multidisciplinary approach, consisting of vigorous chest physiotherapy, mucolytics, antibiotics to treat chest infections, pancreatic enzyme replacement (Creon), and in some cases heart–lung transplantation may be an option in the final stages of the disease. Life expectancy is markedly reduced with a median survival of around 35 years. End-stage lung disease is the principal cause of death.

Gene therapy is not a well-established treatment option and is still best confined to clinical trials. The main problems that have been encountered in the application of gene therapy to clinical practice concern the targeting of vectors to specific sites and integration into the genome.

92 E Affects the intrinsic, rather than the extrinsic, pathway for blood coagulation

Haemophilia A is a sex-linked (X-linked recessive) disorder that results in a reduction in the amount or activity of the clotting factor, factor VIII, a member of the intrinsic pathway. As the inheritance pattern is X linked the disorder primarily affects males, because females who carry the affected gene usually do not have bleeding manifestations.

Clinically there is a tendency towards easy bruising and haemorrhage after trauma or operative procedures. In addition, spontaneous haemorrhages are frequently encountered in regions of the body normally subject to trauma, particularly the joints (haemarthroses).

Factor IX deficiency is known as haemophilia B (or Christmas disease) and is clinically indistinguishable from haemophilia A. Treatment of haemophilia A includes clotting factor replacement with recombinant factor VIII. The continued presence of this devastating disease throughout history may be explained by the protective effect against ischaemic heart disease in haemophilia carriers (by reducing the 'stickiness' of the blood – a similar effect to aspirin).

93 ▶ D It is more common in regions of the world where malaria is endemic

Sickle cell anaemia is an autosomal recessive condition, caused by a single base change in the DNA coding for the amino acid in position 6 of the β-chain of haemoglobin (adenine is replaced by thymine). This leads to an amino acid change from glutamic acid to valine.

The resultant haemoglobin, HbS, has abnormal physiochemical properties that lead to sickling of red blood cells and sickle cell disease. Homozygosity at the sickle cell locus is known as sickle cell anaemia, whereas heterozygosity at the same locus is known as the sickle cell trait. Where malaria is endemic, as many as 30% of black Africans are heterozygous. This frequency may be related in part to the slight protection against *Plasmodium falciparum* afforded by HbS.

Clinical manifestations do not occur until around 3–6 months after birth, when the main switch from fetal to adult haemoglobin occurs (fetal haemoglobin does not contain haemoglobin β-chains). Clinical manifestations relate to the sickling of red blood cells as a result of the production of a structurally abnormal haemoglobin. This includes haemolysis (the average red cell survival is shortened from the normal 120 days to about 20 days) and occlusion of small blood vessels, resulting in ischaemic tissue damage (so-called painful vaso-occlusive crises). The latter crises are precipitated by factors such as infection, acidosis, dehydration and hypoxia. Homozygotes sickle at $P(o_2)$ levels of 5–6 kPa (ie normal venous blood) and thus sickling takes place all the time. Heterozygotes sickle at $P(o_2)$ levels of 2.5–4 kPa and therefore sickle only at extremely low oxygen tensions.

The spleen is enlarged in infancy and childhood, as a result of extramedullary haematopoiesis, but later is often reduced in size (autosplenectomy) as a result of erythrostasis within the spleen, leading to thrombosis, autoinfarction or at least marked tissue hypoxia. Therefore, one should not expect to find a palpable spleen on examining an adult with sickle cell anaemia.

 94 **C Defective haem synthesis results in porphyria**

Sickle cell disease is caused by the production of abnormal globin and thalassaemia by the decreased production of normal globin.

Both sickle cell disease and thalassaemia seemingly developed as a form of carrier resistance against malaria, and as such are widespread in areas profoundly affected by malaria, predominantly Africa, south-east Asia, the Mediterranean and the Middle East.

The porphyrias are a group of genetic diseases caused by errors in the pathway of haem biosynthesis, resulting in the toxic accumulation of porphyrin precursors. Interestingly, porphyria has been suggested as an explanation for the origin of vampire and werewolf legends, and is believed to have accounted for the insanity exhibited by King George III, which may have cost Britain the American War of Independence.

Carbon monoxide binds 250 times more avidly to haemoglobin than oxygen, resulting in the formation of carboxyhaemoglobin. The result is a decrease in the oxygen-carrying capacity of the blood. Carbon monoxide is a colourless, odourless and tasteless gas, so poisoning often goes unnoticed. Levels of carboxyhaemoglobin > 50–60% result in death. The treatment is 100% oxygen, which competitively displaces carbon monoxide from the haemoglobin, thereby decreasing the half-life of carboxyhaemoglobin from around 4 h to 30 min.

Cyanide binds more strongly than oxygen to the iron atom present in the enzyme, cytochrome oxidase. This deactivates the enzyme and the final transport of electrons from cytochrome oxidase to oxygen cannot be completed. As a result, oxidative phosphorylation is disrupted, meaning that the cell can no longer produce ATP for energy. Tissues that mainly depend on aerobic respiration, such as the CNS and heart, are particularly affected, rapidly resulting in death.

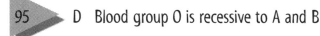

95   D   Blood group O is recessive to A and B

ABO blood groups are inherited in the following manner: blood group O is recessive to both A and B, but A and B exhibit co-dominance. Thus AO or AA = blood group A, BO or BB = blood group B, OO = blood group O, AB = blood group AB.

Blood group O is the most common blood group in the UK population. There is no known evolutionary advantage to being one ABO blood group over another, although people with blood group O are more susceptible to duodenal ulceration than other blood groups, and patients with blood group A are at higher risk of developing gastric carcinoma. Individuals who are Duffy blood group negative, are resistant to *Plasmodium vivax*, because the Duffy antigen acts as a receptor for invasion by the human parasite.

As individuals with blood group AB have no antibodies in their serum, it follows that they are universal recipients. However, they can donate only to other AB individuals. Individuals of blood group O have antibodies present in their serum against blood groups A and B. It therefore follows that they can receive only from other group O individuals. However, they are universal donors because the antibodies are rapidly diluted in the recipient's blood. As blood group O is the universal donor, it is used in emergency situations when there is not enough time to determine the exact blood grouping of the patient.

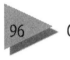

96 **C** **Is associated with berry aneurysms of the circle of Willis**

Adult polycystic kidney disease is one of the most common inherited disorders in humans affecting about 1 in 1000 individuals and accounting for 10% of cases of end-stage renal failure. It is inherited as an autosomal dominant condition with a late-onset mode of presentation. Of cases 85% have been localised to a gene on the short arm of chromosome 16 (*PKD1* gene).

A second gene (*PKD2*), responsible for around 15% cases, has been localised to the long arm of chromosome 4. The corresponding gene products have been named polycystin-1 and polycystin-2, although their exact function is unknown.

Both kidneys are progressively replaced by enlarging cysts that compress and replace the functioning renal parenchyma, leading to renal failure. The condition usually presents in adult life (typically around 40 years of age). When renal failure occurs, it usually progresses to end-stage renal failure at the age of 40–60 years.

Adult polycystic kidney disease is associated with cerebral berry aneurysms (so that death may occur as a result of subarachnoid haemorrhage). Other extrarenal manifestations include liver, pancreatic and splenic cysts.

Section D
Medical
statistics and
epidemiology

Medical statistics and epidemiology
Questions

97 The decline in incidence of serious infections during the nineteenth and twentieth centuries is the result mainly of which of the following?

- ○ A Better sanitation
- ○ B Antibiotics
- ○ C Immunisation programmes
- ○ D A decline in the virulence of organisms
- ○ E Advances in medical science

98 Which of the following changes in disease patterns have occurred in Europe and North America over the past 50 years?

○ A The death rate from lung cancer in females has fallen
○ B The death rate from lung cancer in males has risen in recent years
○ C The numbers infected with HIV are falling
○ D The death rate from suicide has fallen
○ E The death rate from gastric carcinoma has fallen

 99 The most common cause of death from cancer in women is currently:

○ A Ovarian cancer
○ B Breast cancer
○ C Lung cancer
○ D Endometrial cancer
○ E Colon cancer

100 ▶ Which of the following diseases is water borne?

○ A Tuberculosis (TB)

○ B Cholera

○ C Hepatitis C

○ D Plaque

○ E Malaria

101 ▶ With regard to retrospective and prospective studies, which of the following is true?

○ A Prospective studies are also known as case–control studies

○ B Prospective studies allow direct determination of incidence rates

○ C The retrospective approach has the advantage that there is little or no bias

○ D In a prospective study, the cohort consists of people who are found to have the disease in question

○ E The prospective approach is usually used to determine the aetiology of a rare disease

102 Which of the following studies is regarded as the gold standard in epidemiological research?

○ A Cross-sectional study
○ B Case–control study
○ C Case report
○ D Randomised controlled trial
○ E Non-randomised controlled trial

103 You are involved in running a diabetes screening service: 2000 people, aged between 60 and 75 are screened. Both the mean and median random glucose measurements are 9.5 and the standard deviation is 1.4. Which statement is correct?

○ A Five per cent of individuals will have a glucose > 10.9
○ B The distribution is not a normal distribution
○ C Of the individuals 95% will have a blood glucose between 6.7 and 12.3
○ D Of the participants 68% have a blood glucose between 6.7 and 12.3
○ E Of the observations 95% lie between 2 standard errors of the mean

104 Which of the following statements is true?

○ A The standard error provides a measure of the spread of observations around the mean

○ B The standard deviation is equal to the standard error divided by the square root of the sample size

○ C The standard error is generally larger than the standard deviation

○ D In a positively skewed distribution, the median is greater than the mode, but greater then the mean

○ E The mean and standard deviation of a random sample will generally differ from the mean and standard deviation of the true population

105 In a certain trial, the mean ± standard error is 0.5 ± 0.2, with $p < 0.005$. What does this imply?

○ A Of the values 95% lie between 0.1 and 0.9

○ B This difference would have arisen by chance alone less than 1 in 200 times

○ C This difference would have arisen by chance alone less than 1 in 20 000 times

○ D One can be 95% confident that the true population mean lies somewhere within the interval 0.3–0.7

○ E There is a 2.5% chance that the true population mean lies outside the range 0.1–0.9

The following table shows the results for a screening test for pancreatic cancer in 100 people.

| | Disease | |
Test	Positive	Negative
Positive	4	5
Negative	1	90

Which of the following is true?

○ A The positive predictive value is 0.95

○ B The sensitivity is 0.95

○ C The specificity is 0.8

○ D The negative predictive value is 0.99

○ E The sensitivity and specificity depend on the disease prevalence

Medical statistics and epidemiology Answers

 97 ▸ A Better sanitation

The reduced incidence of serious infections (eg typhoid, cholera, TB, smallpox) is mainly the result of improved sanitation. Indeed, sanitation, particularly sewage and the provision of fresh water supplies, has had a much greater impact on the incidence of these diseases than advances in medical science.

Thus, for TB most of the decline in mortality came before the introduction of chemotherapy and the BCG immunisation. Having said that mortality from bacterial infections was much reduced by the advent of antibiotics and immunisations have led to a considerable reduction in incidence of many viral infections. One such success story has been the worldwide eradication of smallpox through a mass immunisation programme. After successful immunisation campaigns the WHO officially declared the total eradication of smallpox in 1979.

Medical statistics and epidemiology – Answers

98   E   The death rate from gastric carcinoma has fallen

ANSWERS

The death rate from lung cancer in women has shown a steep rise since 1955, with no decline in the rate of increase. This may be attributable to the increasing smoking habits of women in modern society. In males the death rate from lung cancer peaked in the mid-1980s and has shown a slight fall since then.

Suicide rates in all countries fall during wartime and were low in the 1950s. Since then they have shown a steady increase in both sexes.

In 1980 the terms 'HIV' and 'AIDS 'did not even exist. However, as of January 2006, just over 25 years after its recognition, the WHO has estimated that 38.6 million people worldwide are HIV positive and more than 25 million people have died of AIDS-related deaths since its recognition, making it one of the most destructive pandemics in recorded history.

Much more mysterious is the downward trend in deaths from stomach carcinoma over the past 50 years. Such trends provide us with valuable information about the aetiology of stomach cancer. This downward trend may be the result of a decrease in some dietary carcinogens. However, the more recent decline may in part be the result of *Helicobacter pylori* eradication therapy because it is now believed that *H. pylori* plays a pivotal role in the development of gastric carcinoma.

MCQs in Applied Basic Sciences for Medical Students: Volume 2

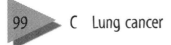

99 C Lung cancer

Currently lung cancer is the most common cause of death from cancer in women, followed by breast cancer and then colorectal cancer. Breast cancer is the most common cancer (in terms of incidence) in women, followed by lung cancer and then colorectal cancer.

The most common cause of death from cancer in men is lung cancer, followed by prostate cancer and then colorectal cancer. In men the most common cancer (in terms of incidence) is prostate cancer, followed by lung and then colorectal cancer.

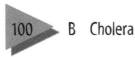

100 B Cholera

Infections, in general, can be transmitted horizontally or vertically, through direct or indirect contact. Vertical transmission occurs when the mother is the source of infection for the fetus.

Example of horizontal routes of transmission:

- air-borne diseases (eg TB), via droplet inhalation/aerosol
- water-borne diseases (eg cholera)
- food-borne diseases (eg dysentery); also known as faecal–oral spread
- blood borne (eg hepatitis C)
- sexual contact (eg HIV)
- oral contact/salivary transfer (eg Epstein–Barr virus)
- vector-borne (ie carried by rats or mosquitoes) diseases (eg plague, malaria)
- infected/contaminated inert objects, or fomites (eg tetanus).

Vertical routes of transmission include:

- transplacental (eg rubella)
- parturition/puerperal (eg ophthalmia neonatorum)
- from breast milk (eg cytomegalovirus or CMV).

101   B   Prospective studies allow direct determination of incidence rates

In a prospective (or cohort) study, exposed and non-exposed individuals are identified and followed up over time to determine the incidence of a specific clinical disease, or event, eg a population of smokers and non-smokers is followed up to provide comparison rates for lung cancer or heart disease. The incidence of a disease is the number of new cases per unit population per unit time.

Cross-sectional studies are like a snapshot in time and measure both exposure and outcome at one time point. They provide information on disease prevalence in a population. Prevalence of a disease is the proportion of a population that exhibits the disease at any one time.

Retrospective (or case–control) studies compare individuals with and without a disease to determine possible associations or risk factors for the disease in question. However, bias may influence the recall of exposure in these studies, especially if possible associations are known (recall bias). In addition, selection bias may impact on the study. A case–control study is relatively easy and inexpensive to conduct because long-term follow-up is not required and this type of study is therefore suitable for studying rare diseases.

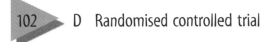

102 ▶ D Randomised controlled trial

Randomised controlled trials form the gold standard in epidemiological research. They resemble cohort studies in many respects, but include the randomisation of participants to exposures. Randomisation is an important part of the study design because it eliminates the effects of selection and confounding biases.

Double blinding or masking (keeping trial participants and investigators oblivious to the assigned intervention) adds to the value of a randomised controlled trial by eliminating the effects of information bias.

Case reports are unreliable because they represent only single cases and do not have a comparison group to allow assessment of associations. However, they are often the first foray into a new disease or area of enquiry. Case–control studies are prone to bias. Cross-sectional studies measure both exposure and outcome simultaneously, and therefore the temporal relationship between the two may be unclear.

ANSWERS

Medical statistics and epidemiology – Answers

103 ▸ C Of the individuals 95% will have a blood glucose between 6.7 and 12.3

The blood glucose values follow a normal (Gaussian) distribution because the mean and median values are equal: 95% fall between 2 standard deviations (not 2 standard errors!) of the mean, ie between 6.7 and 12.3; 2.5% of individuals will have a blood glucose > 12.3, and 2.5% will have a blood glucose < 6.7. It is sometimes easier physically to draw the bell-shaped distribution and mark out the values on it. Of the values 68% lie 1 standard deviation away from the mean; 99% of values lie within 2.6 standard deviations of the mean.

104 ▸ E The mean and standard deviation of a random sample will generally differ from the mean and standard deviation of the true population

The standard error (SE) of the mean measures the variability of a sample statistic (ie mean or proportion) in relation to the true population characteristic (ie how accurate the sample mean is as an estimate of the true population mean). The standard deviation (SD) is a measure of the variability of observations around the mean.

The SE is equal to the SD divided by the square root of the sample size. The SE is therefore generally smaller than the SD. In addition, the SE is smaller when the sample size is larger.

- the mean is the arithmetic average
- the median is the middle value when the values are ranked

- the mode is the value that occurs most often.

In a normal (Gaussian) distribution, the mean = median = mode. In skewed distributions the following three rules apply:

1. The median always lies between the mean and the mode.
2. The mode occurs at the maximum point in a frequency distribution curve.
3. The mean is affected by outliers.

Thus, in a positively skewed distribution: mean > median > mode. In a negatively skewed distribution: mode > median > mean.

105 ▶ **B This difference would have arisen by chance alone less than 1 in 200 times**

Do not confuse the terms 'standard error' and 'standard deviation'. The standard deviation gives a measure of the spread of the distribution. The smaller the SD (or variance), the more tightly grouped the values. If the values are normally distributed, about 95% of values lie within 2 SD of the mean (not standard errors!).

The standard error is a measure of how precisely the sample mean reflects the population mean. It can be used to construct confidence intervals. Typically a 95% confidence interval is quoted, which means that we are 95% certain that the true population mean lies within the interval given by mean ± 1.96 standard errors. In this case the 95% confidence interval is approximately 0.5 ± 0.4 or 0.1–0.9. There is therefore a 5% chance that the true population mean lies outside the range 0.1–0.9.

The *p* value is a probability that derives from statistical significance tests. It takes the value between 0 and 1. Values close to 0 suggest that the null hypothesis is unlikely to be true. The smaller the *p* value, the more significant the result. A significant result is normally taken as p < 0.05 (or 5%), meaning that the difference would have arisen by chance alone less than 1 in 20 times. A *p* value < 0.005 (or 0.5%) is highly significant, meaning that the difference would have arisen by chance alone less than 1 in 200 times.

106 ▶ D The negative predictive value is 0.99

The sensitivity indicates how sensitive the test is at picking up those people who have the disease and is equal to the number of people who are both disease positive and test positive divided by the number who are disease positive. In this example, it is 4/5. The specificity indicates how good the test is at picking up those people who do not have the disease and is equal to the number of people who are both disease negative and test negative divided by the number of people who are disease negative. In this example it is 90/95.

The positive predictive value estimates the probability that an individual who has a positive test truly has the disease – in this example 4/9. The negative predictive value estimates the probability that a individual who has a negative test truly does not have the disease – 90/91. The sensitivity and specificity are independent of disease prevalence.

Index

ABO blood groups 95
acarbose 72
acetazolamide 73
acetylcholine 70
acute phase response 10
adaptive immunity 1
adenine 83
adult polycystic kidney disease 96
AIDS 22, 98
allergic rhinitis 14
alpha-adrenoceptor blockers 71
Alzheimer's disease 89
amino acids 81
amiodarone 76
amyloidosis 51, 52
anaphylaxis 14
anaplasia 31
anergy 1
angiogenesis 40
angiosarcoma 41
angiotensin-converting enzyme
    inhibitors 71
angiotensin II receptor antago-
    nists 71
antacids 69
antiarrhythmics 76
antibiotics 74
antibodies 4
    humoral 13
    see also immunoglobulins
antibody-antigen complexes 13
anticipation 90
antiemetics 66

antigenic variation 22
antigen-presenting cells 6
antihypertensives 71
apoptosis 35, 49
apoptotic bodies 49
Arthus reaction 13
asbestos exposure 46
aspirin 11, 64, 65, 67
asthma 78
astrocytoma 37, 47
atherosclerosis 62
atropine 70
autoantigens 16
autoimmune disease 16
autoimmunity 12
autosomal dominant disorders 85
autosomal recessive disease 86,
    87

bacteria 17
Barrett's oesophagus 33
basic fibroblast growth factor 40
benzatropine 77
beta-adrenoceptor blockers 71,
    76
bladder carcinoma 41
blood glucose 103
blood groups 85
B lymphocytes 3, 9
bone tumours 48
bovine spongiform
    encephalopathy 30
brain tumours 47

BRCA-1 43
breast carcinoma 37, 48, 99
bromocriptine 77
bronchial carcinoma 37
Burkitt's lymphoma 42

cabergoline 77
calcium channel blockers 71, 76
calor 50
cancer cachexia 19
carbon monoxide 94
carcinogens 41
carcinoma 31, 36, 37, 38
carcinoma *in situ* 31
case-control studies 101
caseous necrosis 56
case reports 102
CD4 antigen 75
CD4 T cells 9
CD8 T cells 9
cell cycle 82
cell division 55
central nervous system 55
cephalosporins 74
cholera 20
cholera toxin 20
cholesterol 62, 75
Christmas disease 86, 92
chromosome disorders 88, 89
cimetidine 69
clinical trials 102
clostridia 26
Clostridium botulinum 26
Clostridium difficile 26
Clostridium perfringens 26
Clostridium tetani 26
Clostridium welchii 26
clot 59

coagulative necrosis 56
cohort studies 101
colestyramine 75
colorectal cancer 99
colour blindness 86
complement system 8
    alternative pathway 8
    classic pathway 8
C-reactive protein 10
Creutzfeldt-Jakob disease 30
Crohn's disease 53
cyanide 94
cyclo-oxygenase 11, 64
cystic fibrosis 86, 91
cytochrome oxidase 94
cytokines 10, 11, 12
cytology 35
cytosine 83
cytotoxic T cells 9

delayed type hypersensitivity 13
depolarising neuromuscular
    blockers 70
diabetes mellitus 62
diarrhoea, rice-water 20
diltiazem 76
diuretics 71, 73
DNA amplification 80
DNA oncogenic viruses 42
DNA structure 83
dolor 50
L-dopa 77
dopamine antagonists 66
Down syndrome 89
dysplasia 31

embolus 59
endothelial cells 54

endotoxins 17
enhancers 84
entacapone 77
epinephrine 63
Epstein-Barr virus 42
ethambutol 25
eukaryotes 81
eukaryotic cells 79
exons 84

factor IX deficiency 86, 92
fat necrosis 56
fever 11
fibrates 75
fibrillin 90
fibrinogen 67
fibrinoid necrosis 56
fibrinolytics 67
fibroblasts 54
fibrosis 54
flatworms 29
flecainide 76
fluor 50
follicular dendritic cells 3
functio laesa 50
fungi 17
furosemide 73

gangrene 57
gastric carcinoma 98
gastric hyperacidity 69
gastric mucosa 65
gaussian distribution 103, 104
gene transcription 84
Ghon focus 25
glibenclamide 72
gliclazide 72
glioblastoma multiforme 37

gliosis 54
Golgi apparatus 79
gompertzian kinetics 39
Goodpasture's syndrome 13
Gram-negative bacteria 17
Gram-positive bacteria 17
granulation tissue 54
granuloma 24
granulomatous inflammation 53
Graves' disease 13
guanethidine 70
guanine 83
Guthrie test 86, 87

H_2-receptor antagonists 69
haemarthroses 92
haemoglobin 93
haemophilia A 86, 92
haemophilia B 86, 92
Haemophilus influenzae 18
Helicobacter pylori 19, 42, 98
heparin 58
hepatitis A 21
hepatitis B 21
    immunisation 21
histamine 1
histology 35
HIV 9, 22, 98
Hodgkin's disease 42
humoral antibodies 13
Huntington's disease 86, 90
hyperacute rejection 15
hyperglycaemia 72
hyperplasia 31
hyperpyrexia 11
hypersensitivity 13
    type I 13, 14
    type II 13, 14

type III 13, 14
type IV 13, 14
type V 13, 14
hypertension 62
hypertrophy 31
hypovolaemia 60

immune evasion 18
immune pathology 21
immunoglobulins 5
   IgA 5
   IgG 5
   IgM antibodies 5
immunologically privileged sites
   12
infarction 60
infections
   horizontal transmission 100
   reduced incidence 97
   vertical transmission 100
inflammation
   acute 1, 2, 50, 51
   chronic 52
   granulomatous 53
   outcomes 51
influenza 23
innate immunity 1, 10
interleukins 10
ipratropium 78
ischaemia 59, 60
isoniazid 25

karyolysis 35
karyorrhexis 35
Klinefelter syndrome 88
Knudson's two-hit hypothesis 45
kuru 30

Langerhans' dendritic cells 3, 12
Langhans' giant cells 53
lansoprazole 69
latex allergy 14
leiomyosarcoma 32
leukotriene receptor antagonists
   78
lidocaine 76
lipoprotein 75
liposarcoma 32
liquefactive necrosis 56
local anaesthetics 63
lung cancer 46, 48
   in women 98, 99
lymphadenopathy 3
lymph nodes 3
lymphocytes see B lymphocytes; T
   lymphocytes
lymphoma 32
lysosomes 79
lysozyme 1, 2

macrolides 74
macrophages 1, 2, 54
major histocompatibility complex
   6, 7
   class I 7
   class II 7
malaria 27
   parasite life cycle 28
malignant hyperthermia 70
Marfan syndrome 86
mast cells 1
   degranulation 13
meiosis 82
melanoma 37
meningioma 47
mesothelioma 41

metabolic disorders 86
metaplasia 31, 33
metastasis 36
metazoa 29
metformin 72
micro-organisms 17
    oncogenic 42
misoprostol 69
mitochondria 79
mitosis 82
molecular mimicry 16
montelukast 78
mosquitoes 27, 28
motion sickness 66
mRNA 81
mucoviscidosis *see* cystic fibrosis
multiple myeloma 4, 48
multiple sclerosis 12
myasthenia gravis 70
mycobacteria 2, 24, 25
Mycobacterium tuberculosis 24, 25
myocardial infarction 61

NADPH oxidase 2
nasopharyngeal carcinoma 42
natural killer cells 1
necrosis 35, 56, 57, 60
Neisseria meningitidis 18
neoplasia 31
neurofibromatosis 86
neuromuscular blockers 70
neutrophils 1, 2, 52
nickel sensitivity 13
nicotinic acid 75
non-depolarising neuromuscular
    blockers 70
non-steroidal anti-inflammatory
    drugs 69

normal (gaussian) distribution
    103, 104
northern blotting 80
null hypothesis 105

omeprazole 69
oncogenes 43, 82
opioids 68
opsonisation 8
oral rehydration therapy 20

p53 44
paraneoplastic syndromes 46
parasites 17
Parkinson's disease 77
penicillins 74
peptic ulcer disease 65
pergolide 77
phagocytes 1
phagocytosis 13
phenylketonuria 86, 87
plaque 62
Plasmodium falciparum 27, 28
Plasmodium malariae 27, 28
Plasmodium ovale 27, 28
Plasmodium vivax 27, 28
polymerase chain reaction 80
porphyria 94
positive predictive value 106
potassium-sparing diuretics 73
praziquantel 29
prions 30
procainamide 76
prokaryotes 81
prokaryotic cells 79
promoters 84
prospective (cohort) studies 101
prostaglandins 11, 64, 65

prostate cancer 48, 99
proteasomes 79
proton pump inhibitors 65, 69
proto-oncogenes 43
protozoa 17, 29
p value 105
pyknosis 35
pyrazinamide 25
pyridoxine 25

randomised controlled trials 102
ranitidine 69
Rb-1 44, 45
reactive hyperplasia 3
renal cell carcinoma 37, 48
respiratory burst 2
retinoblastoma 45
retrospective (case-control) studies 101
rhabdomyosarcoma 32
rifampicin 25
RNA oncogenic viruses 42
ropinirole 77
rosiglitazone 72
rubor 50

salbutamol 78
salmeterol 78
sanitation 97
sarcoidosis 53
sarcoma 32, 36, 38
schisotosomiasis 29
Schistosoma haematobium 29, 42
Schistosoma japonicum 29
Schistosoma mansoni 29
scoline apnoea 70
scrapie 30
scrotal (Pott's) cancer 41

selegiline 77
sensitivity 106
septic shock 19
serum sickness 13
sickle cell anaemia 93, 94
silencers 84
skewed distribution 104
skin carcinoma 41
smallpox, eradication of 97
smoking 46, 62
smooth endoplasmic reticulum 79
sodium cromoglicate 78
somatic hypermutation 4
sotalol 76
Southern blotting 80
specificity 106
spleen 18
splenomegaly 93
squamous metaplasia 33
standard deviation 103, 105
standard error 105
standard error of the mean 104
statins 75
steroids 78
Streptococcus pneumoniae 18
streptokinase 67
suicide rate 98
sulphonylureas 72
suxamethonium 70
systemic lupus erythematosus 13

tetanospasmin 26
tetanus 26
thalassaemia 94
T helper cells 9, 75
theophylline 78
thiazide diuretics 73

thrombocytopenia 58
thrombolytics 67
thromboxane A2 64
thrombus 58, 59
thymine 83
thyroid cancer 48
tissue repair 54
T lymphocytes 3, 9
transcription 81
translation 81
transplant rejection 15
trisomy 21 89
tuberculosis 2, 24, 25, 53
   reduced mortality 97
tumour necrosis factor-α 10
tumours 31
   benign 32, 34
   growth 39, 40
   malignant 32, 34
tumour-suppressor genes 44
Turner syndrome 88

urease 19

vascular endothelial growth factor
   40
vasoconstriction 63
vasopressin 73
Vaughan Williams' classification 76
verapamil 76
vertical transmission 100
Vibrio cholerae 20
Virchow's triad 58
viruses 17, 23
   oncogenic 42
von Recklinghausen's disease 86

warfarin 58, 67
western blotting 80
wound healing 54

xanthines 78

Zahn's lines 59
Ziehl–Neelsen stain 25

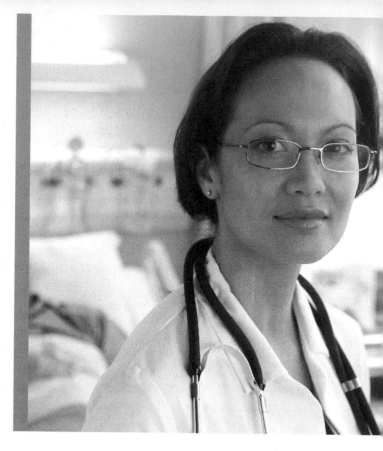

See a specialist

MLP Private Finance plc is part of the MLP Group, one of the leading Independent Financial Advisers in Europe. We specialise in financial planning and wealth management for professionals, and as such our services are tailored to the particular needs of the medical field. MLP provides quality independent advice which means we recommend the most suitable products, plans and funds from the entire marketplace to meet your specific needs and objectives.

We offer financial solutions for: Protection | Insurance | Investments | Savings | Retirement Planning | Mortgages. For more information, contact us on 0845 30 10 999 or info@mlpuk.co.uk or simply visit www.mlp-plc.co.uk.

MLP is the exclusive sponsor of PasTest Undergraduate Finals Revision Courses

MLP Private Finance plc is authorised and regulated by the Financial Services Authority.

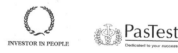

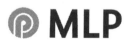